W9-BUN-278

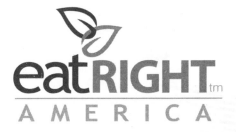

NUTRITARIAN HANDBOOK
AND ANDI FOOD SCORING GUIDE

OTHER BOOKS BY
Joel Fuhrman, M.D.

Eat to Live–
The Revolutionary Formula for
Fast and Sustained Weight Loss

Cholesterol Protection For Life–
Lower Your Cholesterol Safely and Permanently

Disease-Proof Your Child–
Feeding Kids Right

Fasting and Eating for Health–
A Medical Doctor's Program for Conquering Disease

Eat For Health–
The Original High-Nutrient-Density Program
to Achieve Ideal Weight and Superior Health
Two-Book Set

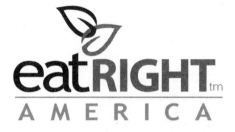

eatRIGHT tm
A M E R I C A

Nutritarian Handbook
AND ANDI FOOD SCORING GUIDE

JOEL FUHRMAN, M.D.

Nutritional Excellence, LLC

COPYRIGHT 2010 BY NUTRITIONAL EXCELLENCE, LLC
All Rights Reserved

No part of this book may be reproduced in any form or by any
electronic or mechanical means, including information storage and
retrieval systems, without permission in writing from the copyright
holder, except by a reviewer who may quote brief passages in a review.

For information, contact:
Nutritional Excellence, LLC
(877) 525-8384
www.EatRightAmerica.com/Handbook

Printed in the United States of America
ISBN-13: 978-0-9825541-0-4
Library of Congress Control Number: 2007931556

Publisher's Note:
Keep in mind that results vary from person to person. Some people
have a medical history and/or condition that may warrant individual-
ized recommendation and, in some cases, drugs and even surgery. Do
not start, stop, or change medication without professional medical
advice, and do not change your diet if you are ill or on medication,
except under the supervision of a competent physician. Neither this,
nor any other book, is intended to take the place of personalized
medical care or treatment.

For reasons of privacy, the names of patients have been changed.

Book Design — Creative Syndicate, Inc.

*This book is dedicated to our friends at
Whole Foods Market whose passion for health
and dedication to their Team Members and customers
have been truly inspirational*

ENJOY
A
WHOLE
LIFE!

CONTENTS

FOREWORD

Eat Right, America! We have all heard the phrase, "you are what you eat," but very few Americans take it to heart. That is why the average weight of an American adult has increased 24 pounds over the past thirty years! Even worse, our miserable eating habits have filtered down to our children who, according to the Centers for Disease Control and Prevention (CDC), will be the first generation in our nation's history NOT to live as long as their parents. It's disgraceful that a nation spending over $2 trillion each year on health care has children developing life-shortening diseases before the age of ten.

America is the richest nation on the face of the earth with the most abundant supply of affordable healthy food, yet according to the USDA less than 5% of Americans get their minimum daily requirement of nutrients. This is when 84% of all health care spending ($1.8 trillion) is directly attributed to our diet! The U.S. Surgeon General called the obesity crisis; "a greater threat to our economy than terrorism." When it comes to health, our nation scores a "D" for disease ridden.

- According to the World Health Organization, America is the fattest nation on the face of the earth. Two-thirds of us are overweight and one-third is obese.

- The CDC estimates half of all children will be overweight by the end of 2010.

- Nearly two-thirds (64%) of all households have at least one member living with a diet related chronic illness, 19% of whom are children.

- Diabetes incidence is growing at epidemic rates. It is estimated that 27 million Americans have diabetes, and another 54 million Americans have pre-diabetes (meaning they will most likely develop diabetes within the next five years).

- Adult Type II Onset Diabetes is now developing in children and has increased 48% in just the past five-years. The CDC predicts one-third of all children born in the year 2000 will develop diabetes before they turn forty. Statistics tell us that these unfortunate children will live fourteen (14) fewer years and will have twenty-two (22) fewer years of quality life.

- 70% of twelve-year olds have already developed signs of heart disease.

Keep this in mind the next time you consider feeding your kids McDonald's, Pizza Hut, Wendy's or some other sodium and fat saturated fast food.

I first heard these startling facts about our children's future while attending a technology conference in the UK. As the father of two beautiful girls, Nancy (12) and Claire (9), needless to say I was shocked. While delicious fruits and vegetables were always around, foods such as chicken nuggets, French fries, soda, chips, fried foods, processed meats, fast food, pizza and many other harmful foods were making their way into my children's diet. While my wife and I began to immediately implement healthier eating habits at home, I knew this was not enough.

Back in 2005, I was the founder and CEO of a technology company that analyzed supermarket frequent shopper card data. My company specialized in identifying families with children so brands like Coca-cola, Nabisco, Frito-Lay and others could deliver money saving coupons for products that were causing many of our nation's health issues. So I began reading everything I could to identify what was causing our nation's problems. What I quickly discovered was that Americans were malnourished and as a result were becoming addicted to foods. I found that the Standard America Diet (SAD) consists of 63% processed foods (empty calories), 25% meat and dairy and only 12%

healthy fruits, vegetables and whole grains. It was easy to see why so many people are overweight and sick. As a nation, we have simply stopped eating REAL FOOD. We have become a nation living on "manufactured foods" full of chemicals and substances that can't even be pronounced. So, in 2005, I closed my company, sold our beautiful home in New Canaan, CT to fund the necessary research, and created Eat Right America.

OUR MISSION:
Deliver the information, programs and support families need to enjoy a whole life.

Not knowing much about nutrition and with the 2005 Pyramid being introduced, I thought it would be a good idea to utilize the technologies I had created to help bring the USDA's Food Pyramid to life. What a mistake. Through months of research, I found that the USDA Food Pyramid is actually at the heart of America's healthcare problems. If there was ever a case of the fox watching the hen house, it is the United States Department of Agriculture. Since the introduction of the first Graphic Food Pyramid in 1992, Americans have gained more weight than any other period in our nation's history. What I discovered is that nearly every influential person within the USDA had come from the meat, dairy or poultry industry. As recently as 2000, six of the eleven board members including the chairman had financial ties to the food industry. As long ago as

1990, proposed changes to the USDA dietary guidelines would have greatly reduced the recommended levels of meat and dairy—a leading cause of heart disease. However, by the time lobbyists and special interests were through, the recommended levels remained alarmingly high and heart disease continues to flourish. I had to abandon this strategy and continue my quest to discover the healthiest dietary lifestyle.

Believing Americans needed to get more nutrients into their diet, in 2005 and 2006, Eat Right America sponsored research with Tufts Friedman School of Nutrition and Yale University to create algorithms that would score foods based on their nutrient density. Hundreds of research studies had proven that a **high-nutrient diet** would both prevent and reverse chronic diseases—while enabling the body to lose weight and keep it off. It was during this period that I read a book called *Eat To Live* by Joel Fuhrman MD. In Chapter One, Dr. Fuhrman talked about an overfed yet undernourished nation. In Chapter Two, he described how Americans are digging their graves with a knife and a fork. Later, he described a simple yet powerful principle: H=N/C (Health=Nutrients over Calories.) After speaking with Dr. Fuhrman, I found that he was a physician who for the past fifteen years had actually applied these nutritional principles to thousands of patients with unbelievable results. In countless cases, people were literally cured of Type II diabetes, heart disease and a host of other illnesses while losing more weight than they ever would have imagined on a typical calorie-counting or popular fad diet. In March 2007, Dr. Fuhrman joined Eat Right America as our Chief Medical Officer and we began working on the programs that would bring a solution to America's healthcare crisis. His book *Eat For Health* soon followed, opening up the possibility of change to thousands more food addicted people.

What was most exciting was how Dr. Fuhrman analyzed each patient's risk factors and eating behavior to determine where they were nutrient deficient and at risk. He would then prescribe a personalized eating plan specifically designed to provide the nutritional and dietary guidance they would need to reverse their chronic condition or effectively lose weight. Dr. Fuhrman and I spent the next two years developing an on-line, automated version that delivers the customized nutritional information people need to possibly save their lives - the program is available at www.eatrightamerica.com/handbook. ERA's Nutrition Prescription is already serving the needs of thousands of families around the globe and is now available through Whole Foods Markets where their remarkable CEO John Mackey has re-focused his company on health.

The good news is that there is still time. Research has proven that a properly nourished body can easily repair itself and be cured of diseases. Type II Diabetics can become insulin free, sometimes in a matter of weeks. People with heart disease can literally be cured.

Migraines disappear. Weight falls off and stays there. The research and information represented in this little book should give you hope for a healthier more productive future, but it is up to you. America is an all-you-can-eat buffet. We simply need to make healthier (smarter) choices. As the first order of business, commit yourself to just eating food. In other words, if it wasn't on the supermarket shelf 100-years ago, lay off!

The Eat Right America Nutritarian Handbook will also explain how eating a diet that is rich in "micronutrients" will enable you to:

- Conquer food addictions and cravings that cause over-eating.
- Easily lose weight and keep it off regardless of how many diets have failed you in the past.
- Prevent and reverse diabetes, heart disease and almost every other diet related chronic illness.
- Have more energy.
- Do away with depression and anxiety.
- Look and feel years younger.
- Eliminate headaches.
- Reduce and then even eliminate your medications.
- Know that you are giving your children the best opportunity to live a long, healthy life.

They say nothing is as powerful as an idea whose time has come. The time is now for all of us to implement the ONLY healthcare that will ever solve our nation's health problems, or yours. It's called "Self-Care" and it's up to you.

So… *Eat Right, America!*

God Bless You and Be Well.

Kevin J. Leville
Founder and CEO
EAT RIGHT AMERICA

INTRODUCTION

No one wants to have a heart attack, suffer a debilitating stroke or develop cancer. But lots of people die from these conditions every day… unnecessarily.

Nutritional science has made dramatic advances in recent years. The overwhelming accumulation of scientific knowledge points to a dramatic conclusion—the majority of diseases plaguing Americans are preventable. Using the information gleaned from scientific studies, it is now possible to formulate a few simple diet and lifestyle principles that can save you years of suffering and premature death. You have an unprecedented opportunity in human history to live healthier and longer than ever before.

But living healthier and longer comes at a price.

How much would it be worth to you for a guarantee that you would never have a heart attack or a stroke? What would it be worth to you to see your children and grandchildren grow healthfully and happily? What would you be willing to pay for the assurance that you would not leave your spouse or your children all alone?

Fortunately, the expenditure is infinitely affordable—little more than the effort needed to establish new, more healthful eating habits.

Everything in this book is supported by the preponderance of evidence from scientific studies. Still, the facts and guidelines contained herein will astound most physicians. Although the research is readily available for all to see, most physicians still have no idea that food can be your most powerful artillery in the fight against the major illnesses that plague Americans.

CHAPTER ONE

AMERICA'S HEALTH CRISIS AND YOU

Americans are digging their graves with their knives and forks. It is not news that Americans are sickly and fat. Almost everybody knows modern America is in the midst of an all-you-can eat food fest that has us literally busting at the seams. We are not only eating ourselves into sickness and premature death, but we also have a health care crisis with upward spiraling medical care costs. It is weighing down our economy, sending jobs overseas and pulling our nation into an economic downspin that is almost impossible to recover from.

The economic costs of heart disease and other diet-related chronic diseases are staggering. Health care costs increased over 50 percent between 2000 and 2005 and now our nation's medical costs exceed 2.4 trillion, over 4 times the amount spent on national defense.[1] These out-of-control costs play an important role in business failures, bankruptcies and loss of jobs. More than 25 percent of the defaults on mortgages and rentals are the result of medical debt.

Our health system relies on an ever-expanding arsenal of medications, tests and procedures that fail to address the *root cause* of our escalating ill health—the way we choose to eat and live. In America, we have attempted to solve our dietary-caused health woes with the development of multiple medications for diabetes, hypertension and cholesterol-lowering as well as heart procedures and surgeries at a dramatic expense. We have been led to believe that drugs and doctors save lives, but the statistics show otherwise; lifespan is not significantly enhanced by the vast majority of medical interventions.

The Obesity Epidemic

Nutritionally-caused disease is now the largest cause of death throughout the world and for the first time globally, the number of overweight individuals rivals the numbers of those who are underweight. In recent years, the growth of processed foods, convenience foods and fast foods has

4

supplied high calorie foods with little nutrients to feed a relatively sedentary society.

In all regions, obesity appears to escalate as income increases and as fast food and processed foods become available. Nowhere has this problem become as large as in America where we have the biggest waistline in the world. In the United States, being overweight is the norm and almost all adults eventually get put on medications for their heart, diabetes, cholesterol or blood pressure.

The number of obese Americans is higher than the number of those who smoke, use illegal drugs or suffer from other physical ailments. Obesity is a major risk factor associated with highly prevalent and serious diseases, such as heart disease, cancer and diabetes and the diet-style that creates these diseases fuels out-of-control medical costs.

The average woman in America today weighs 40 pounds more than women did 100 years ago and has a considerably higher rate of heart attack, strokes and breast cancer to show for it. The rate of sudden cardiac death for the average American male has quadrupled in the past 100 years, and his risk of heart attack is ten times higher. Both sexes, on average, are 30 pounds heavier today than they were in the 1960's. But it is not all about weight. It is much worse than that.

Health Complications of Obesity

- Increased overall mortality
- Adult onset diabetes
- Hypertension
- Degenerative arthritis
- Coronary artery disease
- Obstructive sleep apnea
- Gallstones
- Fatty infiltration of liver
- Restrictive lung disease
- Cancer

Poor Nutrition Everywhere

In the 20th century, processed foods became increasingly prevalent in the average American diet. The consumption of fresh produce and whole grains plummeted while the consumption of animal products increased. As a result, Americans now consume far more calories, fat, cholesterol, refined sugar, animal protein, sodium, white flour and far less fiber and plant-derived nutrients than is healthful. Obesity, diabetes, heart disease and cancer have skyrocketed.

CHANGE IN FOOD CONSUMPTION IN THE LAST 100 YEARS IN THE UNITED STATES

	1900	2000
Sugar	5 lbs/year	170 lbs/year
Soft drinks	0	53 gallons/year
Oils	4 lbs/year	74 lbs/year
Cheese	2 lbs/year	30 lbs/year
Meat	140 lbs/year	200 lbs/year
Homegrown Produce	131 lbs/year	11 pounds/year
Calories	2100	2757

Our society has evolved to a level of economic sophistication that allows us to eat ourselves to death. A diet centered on milk, cheese, pasta, bread, fried foods, sugar-filled snacks and drinks lays the groundwork for obesity, cancer, heart disease, diabetes and autoimmune illnesses. It is not solely that these foods are harmful; it is also what we are not eating that is causing the problem. What we are not eating is enough nutrient-rich foods.

When you calculate all the calories consumed from the Standard American Diet, you find that the calories coming from the most health-promoting foods, such as fresh fruit, vegetables, beans, raw nuts, and seeds, are less than ten percent of the total caloric intake. This dangerously low intake of unrefined plant foods is what guarantees weakened immunity to disease, frequent illnesses and a shorter lifespan. We will never win the war on cancer, heart disease, diabetes, autoimmune diseases and other degenerative illnesses unless we address this deficiency. Though the American diet has spread all over the world, bringing with it heart disease, cancer and obesity, studies still show that in the populations that eat more fruits and vegetables, the incidences of death from these diseases is dramatically lowered.[2]

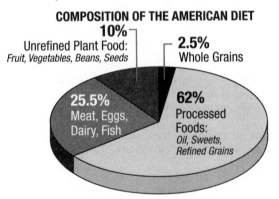

COMPOSITION OF THE AMERICAN DIET

10%
Unrefined Plant Food:
Fruit, Vegetables, Beans, Seeds

2.5%
Whole Grains

25.5%
Meat, Eggs, Dairy, Fish

62%
Processed Foods:
Oil, Sweets, Refined Grains

Heart Disease is Preventable

Heart disease is a much bigger problem than most people think. **Heart attacks and strokes are the cause of death for more than half of all Americans. Yet, heart disease is a relatively new phenomenon in human history and easy to prevent.**

One hundred years ago, heart disease affected only 5% of the population. Today, it affects almost all Americans. Cardiovascular-related deaths have climbed to over 50%. Heart disease kills more people than the next four leading causes of death *combined*. Modern medical techniques and drugs cannot win this war because the true cause of disease is overlooked. Heart disease is caused by inadequate nutrition.

IMPACT OF HEART DISEASE ON AMERICA

- 40 percent of all Americans die of heart attacks
- 58 percent of deaths are related to cardiovascular disease
- 10 percent die of strokes

The tragedy of this is enormous. More than 1.3 million Americans will suffer a heart attack this year, and when you consider that nobody really has to die from a heart- or circulatory-system-related death, it is even more of a tragedy. The disability, suffering and years of life lost are almost totally the result of dietary ignorance. It is not impossible or even difficult to protect yourself; you simply must eat properly. Nothing else can offer such dramatic protection.

9

DEATHS FROM DISEASES OF THE HEART

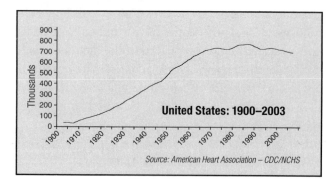

Source: American Heart Association – CDC/NCHS

4 Simple Truths

While America's health crisis is real, you can play an important role in reclaiming your health. Consider these four critical points:

- We are brainwashed into thinking that drugs are the answer to our health problems

- Unhealthy food is addictive

- Foods that don't contain health-promoting micronutrients lead to overeating

- To protect against heart disease, a normal body weight in conjunction with nutritional adequacy is essential

These four simple facts helped create the problems that are killing most Americans. Understanding these simple truths is the solution to what ails America.

The fact is, our bodies' cells need a wide array of nutrients numbering in the thousands to function normally. The human body is designed to be fueled by natural, nutrient-rich plant food. Foods supply not just vitamins and minerals, but thousands of immune-supporting substances called phytochemicals that are essential for our protection against disease.

While science has described these needs, an astonishing 95 percent of Americans do not even meet the Center for Disease Control's (CDC's) minimum nutritional guidelines for the basic vitamins and minerals. Very few people eat healthfully enough to protect themselves against heart disease and cancer in later life.

Why Diets Fail

Low-nutrient eating drives overeating behavior and is the primary cause of obesity, disease and death in the modern world.

Have you ever been on a diet, losing and gaining the same 10, 20 or 30 pounds? Research says that over 95% of all weight lost on a "fad diet" is regained. The biggest problem with most diets is that you are asked to deprive yourself – portion control, low carbs, fewer calories, etc. Deprivation never works and your food cravings return

11

with a vengeance! This unfortunately is the basis of the 'yo-yo' dieting industry. I want you to know that it's not that you have failed a diet; it's that the system (diets, magic pills, surgeries, etc.) has failed you.

My findings, based on my 20 years of experience with over 10,000 patients and thousands of supportive research studies is that a properly nourished body will seek its ideal weight. So instead of 'dieting', I want to show you the foods that provide the nutrition your body needs. **The body has an incredible ability to heal itself and get back in balance when you feed it what it needs. It's that simple!** Your body is like a supercomputer; feed it right and it will keep you fit, lean and healthy.

Enjoy a Whole Life

If you are reading this, you are likely someone who is ready to take control of your health! Some of you have bought this handbook to help you lose weight. I want to assure you that you will lose all the weight that you want, even if diets have failed you in the past. **This is the most effective weight loss plan ever documented in medical literature and the results are permanent,** not temporary. According to a recent medical study, the nutritional program presented here is the most effective way to lose weight, especially if you have a lot of weight to lose. The subjects, followed for two years, lost more weight than the subjects of any other study in medical history, and they kept it off.[3]

More and more, new medical studies are investigating and demonstrating that diets rich in high-nutrient plant foods have a suppressive effect on appetite and are most effective for long-term weight control.[4] The healthiest way to eat is also the most successful way to obtain a favorable weight, if you consider long term results

I am thrilled to be able to work with you and address your weight and diet-related health issues. If you need to lose weight, it will come off quickly and you will never have to diet again. Not only will this program help you reverse many of your weight and health issues, you will learn how to feed your body so it operates at its highest level every day. Your energy levels will be amazing, without relying on artificial stimulants like coffee and sugar. You will sleep better, your skin will look better and you will feel and look younger. In short, your properly nourished body will allow you to live life to the fullest!

I thank you for making an investment in your own health. Your desire to succeed is your foundation for achieving a healthy weight and a long, happy life.

CHAPTER TWO

BECOMING A NUTRITARIAN

Not Your Typical Diet

The journey you are about to take is different from any other you've embarked upon for weight loss and health. Typical diet books usually entail a list of rules and regulations to restrict calories for weight loss. This is a problem, because when the focus is weight loss alone, results are rarely permanent.

The focus in this handbook is on nutrition and *eating right*, which is an undisputed, yet often overlooked critical ingredient to any dietary success. Here, there is no calorie counting, portion-size measuring or weighing involved. In fact, you will eat as much food as you want, and still over time you will become satisfied with fewer calories. Follow the advice in this handbook, and you will lose weight and keep it off—because a properly nourished body will *automatically seek its ideal weight*, without you having to fight the scale or count calories for one more day.

The fundamentals of this eating style are to increase high-nutrient foods in your diet and to 'crowd out' unhealthy low-nutrient foods. What does it mean to crowd-out? It means that as you eat more delicious, high-nutrient foods, you will be reducing your desire for fatty, processed and unhealthy products.

When you change the foods you eat to better meet your nutrient needs, you feel better and it eventually becomes your preferred way of eating. To accomplish this, you will be presented with scientific, logical information that explains the connection between food and your weight and health. This information will help you shed pounds naturally and easily, merely as a side effect of eating so healthfully.

What is a Nutritarian?

When you learn this eating style, you can proudly call yourself a Nutritarian. A Nutritarian is someone who strives to consume and learns to prefer foods that are nutritious. Quite simply, a Nutritarian:

- Eats lots of high-nutrient, natural plant foods: vegetables, fruits, beans, nuts and seeds.

- Eats fewer animal products and chooses healthier options in this food group.

• Eats much less or almost no foods that are completely empty of nutrients or toxic for the body such as: sugar, sweeteners, white flour, processed foods and greasy, fast foods.

The Nutritarian way to health, longevity and weight loss focuses on healthy foods such as green vegetables, other colorful vegetables, fruits, beans, nuts and seeds.

A Nutritarian is someone who learns to trust the amazing power of the body. *If given half a chance, the body will heal itself*—with food as the catalyst, nonetheless. When you learn how to become a Nutritarian, you will arm yourself with the biochemical sustenance that your body needs to be at its ideal weight and to live a healthy, empowered life.

Finally, a Nutritarian lifestyle is an attitude, a mindset, a method that can be followed for a lifetime. As you begin your journey as a Nutritarian, you will be empowered to take control of your own health and life.

Vegetarian, flexitarian or nutritarian

The foundation of the Nutritarian diet is vegetables and other high-nutrient foods, but it does not have to be at the exclusion of all animal foods. To clarify, a vegan diet is one that contains no foods of animal product origin whereas a vegetarian diet may contain some dairy. A vegetarian/vegan diet can be an option for excellent health as long as care is taken to eat healthy, nutrient-rich foods. However, a vegetarian/vegan who lives on processed cereals, white flour products, white rice, white potato and processed soy products is still vulnerable to the weight gain, diseases and many of the other complications resulting from the standard American diet because their diet cannot be considered nutrient-rich.

Being a Nutritarian differs from being a typical vegetarian because the focus isn't on totally excluding animal foods, but on including the high-nutrient foods a body needs to improve health dramatically. A Nutritarian will reduce the level of animal products to a safe level without having to exclude them completely. So a Nutritarian could be a vegan or not. Eating this way makes either option healthful.

The Nutritarian difference
The Nutritarian diet is different because it doesn't require deprivation, starvation or denying your body foods that properly nourish it. It truly is a whole new way of looking at food. This handbook will tell you why nutrient-rich foods are so powerful and will help you learn exactly what to eat and how to incorporate these foods into your diet.

By making these changes, your body will change in amazing and drastic ways. Many people who have adopted the Nutritarian lifestyle have reversed many diet-related diseases such as diabetes, heart disease, chronic fatigue, autoimmune disease and migraines, just to name a few.

The right food can be the most healing 'medicine' you put in your body. And once you grasp the possibilities that can occur from eating this way, your health and life will be changed forever.

Nutritarian Pyramid

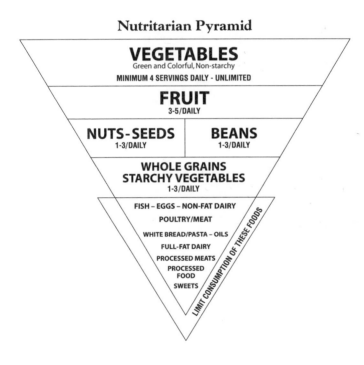

VEGETABLES
Green and Colorful, Non-starchy
MINIMUM 4 SERVINGS DAILY - UNLIMITED

FRUIT
3-5/DAILY

NUTS-SEEDS
1-3/DAILY

BEANS
1-3/DAILY

WHOLE GRAINS
STARCHY VEGETABLES
1-3/DAILY

FISH – EGGS – NON-FAT DAIRY
POULTRY/MEAT
WHITE BREAD/PASTA – OILS
FULL-FAT DAIRY
PROCESSED MEATS
PROCESSED FOOD
SWEETS

LIMIT CONSUMPTION OF THESE FOODS

CHAPTER THREE

THE HEALTH EQUATION

Discovering Nutrients

There are two kinds of nutrients: macronutrients and micronutrients. Macronutrients are protein, carbohydrate, fat (and water). Excluding water, they basically are the three calorie-containing nutrients.

Micronutrients are vitamins, minerals and phytochemicals and are calorie-free. For ideal health, we need to consume both kinds of nutrients, but the American diet contains too many macronutrients and not enough micronutrients.

MACRONUTRIENTS = FAT, CARBOHYDRATE & PROTEIN
CONTAIN CALORIES
SHOULD LIMIT CONSUMPTION

MICRONUTRIENTS = VITAMINS, MINERALS & PHYTOCHEMICALS
DO NOT CONTAIN CALORIES
SHOULD INCREASE CONSUMPTION

Eating foods that are naturally rich in micronutrients is the secret to achieving optimal health. A micronutrient-heavy diet supplies your body with 14 different vitamins, 25 different minerals, and more than 10,000 phytochemicals, which are plant-based chemicals that have profound effects on human cell function and the immune system. Foods that are naturally rich in these nutrients are also rich in fiber and water and are naturally low in calories, meaning they have a low caloric density. These low-calorie, high-nutrient foods provide the ingredients that activate your body's self-healing and self-repairing mechanisms. They are nature's contribution to your health turnaround! The foundational principle of this program is that the right food is your best medicine.

About 80 years ago, when scientists first identified vitamins and minerals, we thought we could have a profound effect on reducing risks of cancer and other life-shortening diseases. When the fortification of foods and the explosion of the supplement industry became a major contributor to America's micronutrient pie, an amazing thing happened. Cancer rates increased for 70 years straight from 1935 to 2005. Certainly, I am not suggesting the ingestion of these micronutrients was primarily to blame, but I am saying that vitamins and minerals alone are definitely not the answer.

We found out about 15 years ago that the major micro-nutrient load in food was NOT vitamins and minerals; it was phytochemicals. Shockingly, natural foods contained many more critical nutritional elements than we had ever imagined. With thousands of nutrients in a strawberry or sprig of broccoli, we found out that nutrient intake was more intricate then we originally thought. With the right assortment of natural foods, these nutrients work harmoniously to protect our body against disease.

Only by including the right variety of nutrient-rich foods can we be offered the dramatic health benefits nature can provide.

The phytochemical revolution

All the different types of nutrients are vital to achieving and maintaining optimal health and nutritional excellence; however, phytochemicals hold a special, elite place in the nutritional landscape. When consistently consumed in adequate quantity and variety, phytochemicals become super-nutrients in your body. They work together to detoxify cancer-causing compounds, deactivate free radicals, protect against radiation damage and enable DNA repair mechanisms.[5] When altered or broken strands of DNA are repaired, it can prevent cancer from developing later in life.

Consuming phytochemicals is not optional. They are essential in human immune-system defenses. Without a wide variety and sufficient amount of phytochemicals from unprocessed plant foods, scientists note that cells age more rapidly and do not retain their innate ability to remove and detoxify waste products and toxic compounds. Low levels of phytochemical-rich produce in our modern diet are largely responsible for the common diseases seen with aging, especially cancer and heart disease. Approximately 85 percent of our population acquires and eventually dies from heart disease, strokes and cancer. This is extremely high compared to other populations around the world and at earlier points in human history. The point is, that we have learned so much from modern nutritional science in the last 15 years, and when applied to our daily life, it works—we can live longer and better with almost no risk of the diseases that plague other Americans..

Let's take heart disease as an example. Heart attacks are extremely rare occurrences in populations that eat a diet rich in protective phytochemicals (from vegetables) such as the Okinawans of Japan, but are omnipresent in populations, such as ours, that eat a diet low in these protective nutrients.[6] Compelling data from numerous population studies shows that a natural, plant-based diet rich in antioxidants and phytochemicals will prevent, arrest and even reverse heart disease.[7]

Our bodies were designed to make use of thousands of plant compounds. When these necessary compounds are missing, we survive because our bodies are adaptable, but over time we lose our powerful potential for wellness and chronic disease develops. We are robbed of living to our fullest potential in good physical, emotional, and mental health. Consumption of healthy foods leads to disease resistance; consumption of unhealthy foods makes us disease-prone.

Eating right enables you to feel your best every day. You may still get sick from a virus, but your body will be in a far better position to defend itself and make a quick and complete recovery. Optimal nutrition enables us to work better, play better, and maintain our youthful vigor as we age gracefully.

The Health Equation

The secret to a long life and disease reversal is to eat a diet lower in calories but higher in nutrients. It is all about nutrient bang per caloric buck.

This important nutritional concept can be presented by a simple mathematical formula, which I call my health equation.

DR. FUHRMAN'S HEALTH EQUATION: H = N/C

Your health is dependent on the nutrient-per-calorie density of your diet.

In this discussion, the word nutrient means micronutrients. Your future health equals nutrient consumption divided by calories. This straightforward mathematical formula is the basis of nutritional science and nutritional healing. This formula essentially states that for you to be in excellent health, your diet must be nutrient-rich, and you must not overeat on calories (or macronutrients). The nutrient density in your body's tissues is proportional to the nutrient density of your diet. By choosing foods and designing our diet with this equation in mind, we realize we must seek out and consume more foods with a high nutrient-per-calorie density and less foods with a low nutrient-per-calorie density.[8]

So in addition to eating more of these micronutrient-rich foods, we need to eat less macronutrients. Every nutritional scientist in the world agrees that moderate caloric restriction in the environment of micronutrient adequacy slows the aging process, prevents the development of chronic diseases and extends lifespan. This has been tested in every species of animal, including primates. There is no controversy that Americans are eating themselves to death with too many calories. To change this we must do three things:

1 - EAT LESS FAT
2 - EAT LESS PROTEIN
3 - EAT LESS CARBOHYDRATE

Even though reduction of calories is valuable, the focus here is different. Because when the fatty foods you eat are high-nutrient fatty foods and the proteins you eat are high nutrient proteins and the carbohydrates you eat are high nutrient carbohydrates, you naturally desire fewer calories.

Natural, whole plant foods are a mixture of fat, carbohydrate and protein; but in their natural state are typically rich in micronutrients, even some not yet discovered.

Simply trying to reduce calories is called dieting, and dieting doesn't work. The reason this program is so successful is because over time, without even trying or noticing it, you will prefer to eat fewer calories. I know that can sound unlikely. Many people think, "Not me," "My body doesn't work that way," or, "It will be a real struggle for me." However, if you follow the plan, it will happen instinctually and almost effortlessly. I have seen it happen to thousands, with all kinds of different backgrounds and eating histories, and I promise, it can happen for you too.

This program will help you lose weight and achieve superior health by eating more nutrient-rich foods and less high-calorie, low-nutrient foods. **It works because the more high-nutrient food you consume, the less low-nutrient food you desire.** Since the desire for these unhealthy foods will naturally diminish, this program is fundamentally about learning how to enjoy eating more high-nutrient food. Foods are nutrient dense when they contain a high level of micronutrients per calorie. Vegetables win the award for the most nutrient-dense foods on the planet. Therefore, as you move forward in your quest for nutritional excellence, you will eat more and more vegetables. Since they contain the most nutrients per calorie, vegetables have the most powerful association with life-extension and protection from heart disease and cancer. It is the only way to achieve your ideal weight permanently.

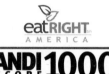

ANDI Scoring System

ANDI stands for **A**ggregate **N**utrient **D**ensity **I**ndex. ANDI brings to life the H = N/C health equation or Health = Nutrients divided by Calories. It is an index that guides you on making every bite count. The "ANDI" Nutrient Score is a rating system that scores foods on a scale of 0–1000. This Index assigns a score to a variety of foods based on adding up all the vitamins and minerals they deliver for each calorie consumed. The most nutrient dense foods score 1000; all other foods are then scored relative to them. Kale, a dark leafy green, scores 1000 while Coke scores 0.6. This is just an easy way to quickly visualize the relative nutrient value of various foods. It demonstrates the nutrient power of green vegetables.

Using the ANDI is simple. It is meant to encourage you to eat more foods that have high numbers and eat larger amounts of these foods because the higher the number, and the greater percentage of those foods in your diet, the better your health.

Because phytochemicals are largely unnamed and unmeasured, these ANDI rankings may underestimate the healthful properties of colorful, natural, plant foods compared to processed foods and animal products. One thing we do know about natural foods is that the foods that contain the highest amount of known nutrients are the same foods that contain the most unknown nutrients. So, even though these rankings may not consider the phytochemical number sufficiently, they are still a reasonable measurement of their content and can be very helpful in giving you an understanding of the value of the food around you.

SAMPLE NUTRIENT/CALORIE DENSITY SCORES

Aggregate Nutrient Density Index* (ANDI)

Kale	1000	Green Pepper	258
Collards	1000	Artichoke	244
Bok Choy	824	Carrots	240
Spinach	739	Asparagus	234
Brussel Sprouts	672	Strawberry	212
Arugula	559	Pomeg. Juice	193
Cabbage	481	Tomato	164
Romaine	389	Blueberries	130
Broccoli	376	Iceberg	110
Cauliflower	295	Orange	109

Lentils	104	Skim Milk	36
Cantaloupe	100	Walnuts	34
Kidney Beans	100	Grapes	31
Sweet Potato	83	White Potato	31
Sunflower Seeds	78	Banana	30
Peach	73	Chicken Breast	27
Apple	72	Eggs	27
Green Peas	70	Peanut Butter	26
Cherries	68	Whole Wheat Bread	25
Flax Seeds	65	Feta Cheese	21
Sesame Seeds	65	Whole Milk	20
Pineapple	64	Ground Beef	20
Edamame	58	White Pasta	18
Oatmeal	53	White Bread	18
Mango	51	Apple Juice	16
Cucumber	50	Swiss Cheese	15
Pistachio Nuts	48	Low Fat Fruit Yogurt	15
Corn	44	Potato Chips	11
Salmon	39	Cheddar Cheese	11
Almonds	38	Vanilla Ice Cream	9
Shrimp	38	Olive Oil	9
Tofu	37	French Fries	7
Avocado	37	Cola	0.6

Many people are surprised that olive oil gets an ANDI of only 9. It is important to recognize that olive oil, like all other oil, has 120 calories per tablespoon. All oil is low nutrient, high calorie food, linked to weight gain. People sabotage their desire to lose weight by using too much oil in their diet.

Matter of Emphasis

Most health authorities today are in agreement that we should add more servings of healthy fruits and vegetables to our diet. I disagree. Thinking about our diet in this fashion doesn't adequately address the problem. Instead of thinking of adding those protective fruits, vegetables, beans, seeds and nuts to our disease-causing diet, **these foods must be the main focus of the diet itself.** This is what makes the Eat Right America program different. Once we understand that concept, then we can add a few servings of foods that are not in this category to the diet each week, and use animal products as condiments or small additions to this naturally nutrient-rich diet.

Chapter Four

Top 30 Foods

Now that you know the secret formula to health is H = N/C (Health = Nutrients/Calories), it's time to start putting it into practice. There are comprehensive lists of nutrient density scores later in this book. But to make it easy for you to find the very best foods, we've listed my Top 30 Super Foods on the following page. These are the best foods in the best categories. For weight loss and improved health, include as many of these foods in your diet as you possibly can.

	NUTRIENT SCORE
1. Collard Greens, Mustard Greens, Turnip Greens	1000
2. Kale	1000
3. Watercress	1000
4. Bok Choy	824
5. Spinach	739
6. Broccoli Rabe	715
7. Chinese/Napa Cabbage	704
8. Brussels Sprouts	672
9. Swiss Chard	670
10. Arugula	559
11. Cabbage	481
12. Romaine Lettuce	389
13. Broccoli	376
14. Red Pepper	366
15. Carrot Juice	344
16. Tomatoes and Tomato Products	164–300
17. Cauliflower	295
18. Strawberries	212
19. Pomegranate Juice	193
20. Blackberries	178
21. Plums	157
22. Raspberries	145
23. Blueberries	130
24. Oranges	109
25. Cantaloupe	100
26. Beans (all varieties)	57–104
27. Seeds: Flaxseed, Sunflower, Sesame	52–78
28. Pistachio Nuts	48
29. Tofu	37
30. Walnuts	34

CHAPTER FIVE

THE
NUTRITION PRESCRIPTION

Three Levels of Nutritional Excellence

I have organized my meal plans into three levels of nutritional excellence. Based on your health needs and current dietary habits, you can choose between three different diet options: Level One, Two or Three. I would like to see everyone reach at least Level Two, although for many, even Level One will represent a significant improvement.

Use my ANDI scores contained in Chapter Four and Eight of this book to help you choose the most nutrient dense foods. You will find sample menus and healthy recipes in Chapters Nine and Ten of this handbook. High nutrient density soups, delicious fruit smoothies and healthy dressings and dips are featured in all my meal plans, however this handbook only gives a sample of the valuable information, menus and recipes available in my more comprehensive *Eat for Health* book and at **www.eatrightamerica.com/handbook**.

I have designed three levels, as an aid to direct people to the level of nutritional excellence they need for their individual health conditions. This does not mean a person should not move to a higher level of excellence if they are comfortable doing so.

TAKE A 28 DAY NUTRITARIAN PLEDGE
Try this nutrient dense eating style for 28 days and you will begin to see a dramatic difference in your health and well being.

All levels require the 28 day pledge to the five cornerstones of healthy eating:

1) A large salad every day

2) At least a half-cup serving of beans/legumes in soup, salad or a dish once daily

3) At least 3 fresh fruits a day

4) At least one ounce of raw nuts and seeds a day

5) At least one large (double-size) serving of steamed green vegetables daily

All the levels require the 28 day pledge to avoid the five most deadly food habits:

1) No barbeque, processed meats or commercial red meat

2) No fried foods

3) No full-fat dairy (cheese, ice cream, butter, whole milk or 2% milk) or trans fat (margarine).

4) No soft drinks, sugar or artificial sweeteners

5) No white flour products

The point is to give your body a real chance to change its biochemistry, build up its nutrient stores and see how much better your life can be when you are well nourished.

Level One

Level One is appropriate for a person who is healthy, thin, physically fit and exercises regularly. They should have no risk factors such as high blood pressure, high cholesterol or a family history of heart disease, stroke or cancer before the age of 75.

Most Americans do have risk factors or a family history of strokes, heart attacks and cancer, and most Americans are overweight. So for most people they should only see

Level One as a temporary stage as they learn about this high nutrient eating style and allow their taste buds to acclimate to high nutrient, healthy eating.

Level One is designed to ease the emotional shock of making such profound dietary improvements. It enables people who feel Level Two or Three is too difficult to revamp their diet at a level that is significant, but not overwhelming. Enjoy this new style of eating, allow your taste preferences to change with time and learn some great healthy recipes. You may soon decide to move on to a higher level. However, I still recommend that the majority of individuals make the commitment to jump right into Level Two or Three because so many people are significantly overweight and have risk factors that need to be addressed with a high level of nutritional excellence immediately. Many are in desperate need of a health makeover and a Level Two or Three diet change is urgent.

In Level One, you eliminate fried foods and substitute fruit-based healthful desserts and whole grains for low nutrient processed snack foods such as salty snacks, candy, ice cream and baked products. Your sodium intake will decrease as you begin to make these dietary changes. Processed foods and restaurant foods contribute 77% of the sodium people consume. Salt from the salt shaker provides 11% and sodium found naturally in food provides the remaining 12%. Select whole grain products like old fashioned oats, wild rice, brown rice, 100% whole grain bread and pasta made with 100% whole grain or bean flour. Eliminate bread and pasta made with refined white flour as pledged for 28 days and hopefully longer.

You also eliminate foods like cheese and butter that are high in saturated fats and your cooking techniques use only a minimal amount of oil. Most Americans consume over 20 servings of animal products weekly. In Level One I recommend only seven servings of animal products per week. These animal products are limited to fish, skinless chicken or turkey, eggs or nonfat dairy products. One serving per week of wild or organic grass fed red meat is allowed.

Level Two

Level Two builds on the positive changes described in Level One. In Level Two, animal products are reduced to four servings weekly and vegetables and beans should start to make up an even larger portion of your total caloric intake. When you incorporate more and more nutrient-rich produce in your diet, you automatically increase your intake of antioxidants, phytochemicals, plant fibers, lignins, and plant sterols. You lower the glycemic index of your diet and the level of saturated fat, salt and other negative elements without having to think about it. Your ability to appreciate the natural flavors of unprocessed, whole foods will improve with time because you lose your dependence on salt and sugar. Add more beans and nuts to your diet to replace animal products.

Try some of the high nutrient dressing and dip recipes in Chapter Ten. They use heart healthy nuts to replace the oils found in traditional dressings and dips.

The Level Two Meal Plan is a good target diet for most people. If you want to lose weight, lower your cholesterol, lower your blood pressure or just live a long healthy life, this Nutritarian diet is the one you should adopt.

Level Three

If you suffer from serious medical conditions like diabetes, heart disease, autoimmune disease or just want to optimize the nutrient density of your diet to slow aging and maximize longevity, I move the level of nutritional excellence up to the max in Level Three. If you suffer from a medical condition that is important to reverse, this is the right prescription for you. If you are on medications and you want to be able to discontinue them as quickly as possible, I recommend following a Level Three diet. It is also the diet-style to follow if you have trouble losing weight, no matter what you do, and want to maximize your results. Level Three is designed for those who want to reverse serious disease or for healthy people who want to push the envelope of human longevity.

This is the diet that I use in my medical practice when people have to reverse serious autoimmune diseases, (such as rheumatoid arthritis or lupus), or when someone has life-threatening heart disease (atherosclerosis). I prescribe it for diabetics who need to lower their blood sugars into the normal range, or to get rid of severe migraines. It delivers the highest level of nutrient density.

This level includes only two servings or less of animal products weekly and maximizes high nutrient density vegetables. Review the Top 30 food list in Chapter Four and the use the ANDI scores in Chapter 8 to select the most nutrient dense foods you can find. Use green smoothies, fresh vegetable juices, healthy soups and lots of raw vegetables to make every calorie count.

At Level Three, you should consume processed foods only rarely. Keep the use of refined fats/oils to a minimum. Nuts and seeds supply essential fats in a much healthier package, with significant health benefits. The recipes in Chapter Ten provide some ideas for incorporating a variety of nutrient dense foods into your diet.

In the following table, I have listed some of the Top foods in the six food categories that should make up 75-80% of your diet. These foods get some of the highest ANDI or nutrient density scores. Below each group, the number of servings suggested to achieve Level One, Two or Three is listed. These amounts should not be seen as rigid requirements, but rather as helpful guidelines. Of course there are many other choices in these categories and I encourage you to try them all.

The Nutrition Prescription:
Recommended Servings of Vegetables, Fruit, Beans & Nuts

COOKED GREEN VEGETABLES

1.5 cups Kale

1.5 cups Mustard, Turnip or Collard Greens

1.5 cups Bok Choy

1.5 cups Broccoli Rabe

1.5 cups Chinese/Napa Cabbage

1.5 cups Spinach

1.5 cups Brussels Sprouts

1.5 cups Swiss Chard

1.5 cups Cabbage

1.5 cups Broccoli

LEVEL ONE	LEVEL TWO	LEVEL THREE
1-2 servings	2-3 servings	2-3 servings

RAW GREEN VEGETABLES

3 cups watercress

5 cups spinach

5 cups romaine lettuce

5 cups arugula

5 cups mixed baby greens

1.5 cups raw Broccoli

1.5 cups cabbage

1.5 cups green pepper

2 cups zucchini

1.5 cups Snow Peas

LEVEL ONE	LEVEL TWO	LEVEL THREE
1 serving	1-2 servings	2-3 servings

NON-GREEN VEGETABLES

1 cup bean/broccoli sprouts

6 radishes

1.5 cups Red Pepper

2 cups Radicchio

1 Turnip

1.5 cups carrots

1.5 cups cauliflower

1 Artichoke

1 Tomato

1.5 cups Butternut Squash

LEVEL ONE	LEVEL TWO	LEVEL THREE
1 serving	1 serving	1 serving

FRUIT

1.5 cups Strawberries

3 Plums

1.5 cups Blueberries

1.5 cups Raspberries

1 Orange

1.5 cups Cantaloupe

2 Kiwis

2.5 cups Watermelon

1 Apple

1.5 cups Cherries

LEVEL ONE	LEVEL TWO	LEVEL THREE
3-5 servings	3-5 servings	3-5 servings

BEANS

1 cup Lentils	1 cup Split Peas
1 cup Red Kidney	1 cup Edamame
1 cup Adzuki Beans	1 cup Chickpeas
1 cup Black Beans	1 cup White Beans
1 cup Pinto Beans	4 oz Tofu

LEVEL ONE	LEVEL TWO	LEVEL THREE
0.5-3 servings	0.5-3 servings	0.5-3 servings

NUTS AND SEEDS

1/4 cup Sunflower Seeds	1/4 cup Pecans
2 Tablespoons Flax Seed	1/4 cup Almonds
1/4 cup Sesame Seeds	1/4 cup Walnuts
1/4 cup Pumpkin Seeds	1/4 cup Cashews
1/4 cup Pistachios	1/4 cup raw nut butter

LEVEL ONE	LEVEL TWO	LEVEL THREE
1-3 servings*	1-3 servings*	1-3 servings*

The amount of nuts and seeds as well as other foods you consume depends on your caloric requirements. If you are trying to lose weight, limit nuts to one serving daily. If you are thin, want to gain weight or need more calories to fuel your athletic activities, then the number of servings may be increased.

Eating enough healthy food is critical to your success as a Nutritarian. You will find that when you eat enough high nutrient food, you no longer desire or even have room for the other foods that used to make up the biggest part of your diet. Processed and refined foods offer little in terms of nutrients and phytochemicals. When you eat them, you are literally throwing away valuable nutrients that could have been put to good use by your body.

Overview of the Three Levels
Recommended Amounts

	LEVEL ONE	LEVEL TWO	LEVEL THREE
VEGETABLES* raw & cooked	3 servings/day	4-6 servings/day	5-7 servings/day
FRUIT*	3-5 servings/day	3-5 servings/day	3-5 servings/day
BEANS	0.5-3 servings/day	0.5-3 servings/day *[one serving = 1/2 to 1 cup]*	0.5-3 servings/day
NUTS & SEEDS	1-3 servings/day	1-3 servings/day ———1 serving/day if trying to lose weight——— *[one serving = 1 ounce or 1/4 cup]*	1-3 servings/day

* *See Nutrient Density Scores in Chapter Eight for suggested serving sizes of specific vegetables and fruit.*

Overview of the Three Levels
Maximum Allowed

	LEVEL ONE	LEVEL TWO	LEVEL THREE
WHOLE GRAIN PRODUCTS/ STARCHY VEGETABLES	4 servings/day or less	4 servings/day or less	3 servings/day or less
	[one serving = 1 slice or 1 cup]		
ANIMAL PRODUCTS**	7 servings/ week or less	4 servings/ week or less	2 servings/ week or less
	[one serving = 4 ounces]		
SODIUM	1600 mg/day or less	1200 mg/day or less	1000 mg/day or less
FATS/OILS substitutes include non-dairy spreads without trans or hydro-genated fats	1 tablespoon of olive oil or acceptable substitute/day	1 tablespoon of olive oil or acceptable substitute/day	1-2 tablespoons/ week

** *Animal Products include: white meat, eggs, low fat dairy. In Levels One and Two up to 1 serving per week of red meat is allowed if it is a wild meat or organic grass fed. ABSOLUTELY NO processed meats, cured meats, BBQ meats or full fat dairy.*

Eat Right America's *Nutrition Prescription*
further customizes the program for you and places you in
one of three levels according to your personal needs.

Go to
www.eatrightamerica.com/handbook
to learn more

My book *Eat for Health* contains more information about
my Nutritarian Eating Plans and resolving the emotional
impediments to dietary change. It features cooking tips,
menus and over 150 healthy recipes.

6

HUNGER AND WEIGHT LOSS

When a heavy coffee drinker completely stops drinking coffee, he feels ill, experiencing headaches and weakness, and even feels nervous and shaky. Fortunately, these symptoms resolve slowly over four to six days. Discomfort after stopping an addictive substance is called withdrawal, and it is significant because it represents detoxification, or a biochemical healing that is accomplished after the substance is withdrawn.

It is nearly impossible to cleanse the body of a harmful substance without experiencing the discomfort of withdrawal. Humans have a tendency to want to avoid discomfort, so they continue the toxic habits to avoid the unpleasant withdrawal symptoms. If we discontinued consuming healthy substances, such as broccoli or spinach, we would not experience discomfort. We would feel nothing. Only unhealthful, toxic substances are addicting, and therefore, these are the only substances that cause discomfort when you stop consuming them. Their addictive potential or discomfort that results from discontinuation is proportional to their toxicity.

Uncomfortable sensations are not always unfavorable. They are very often the signals that repair is under way and the removal of toxins is occurring. Though it may be difficult to adjust to this way of thinking, feeling ill temporarily can be seen as a sign that you are getting well. That cup of coffee may make you feel better temporarily, but any stimulating substance that makes you feel better quickly, or gives you immediate energy, is likely hurtful, not healthful.

The heavy coffee drinker typically feels the worst upon waking up in the morning or when delaying or skipping a meal. The same is true for the many of us who are addicted to toxic foods. The body goes through withdrawal, or detoxification, most strongly when it is not busy digesting food. Eating stops withdrawal because detoxification cannot take place efficiently while food is being consumed and digested. A heavy meal will stop the discomfort, or a cup of coffee will alleviate the symptoms, but the cycle of withdrawal will begin again the minute the caffeine level drops or digestion is finished and the glucose level in the blood starts to go down.

Food Addiction and Weight Gain

When you eat a diet that is based on toxic and addictive foods—such as salty/fried foods, snack foods, and sugary drinks—you set the stage for ill feelings when you are not digesting food. Consuming unhealthy food allows your body to create waste by-products that must be removed by the liver and other organs. Only when digestion ends can the body fully take advantage of the opportunity to circulate and attempt to lower the level of these toxins. By keeping digestion constantly active with eating frequently, or by overeating heavy foods that take a long time to digest we can prevent these ill feelings by curtailing the detoxification process.

Let digestion end and the heightened cycle of detoxification begin, and people will feel queasy, weak or irritable. Eating something restarts digestion and shuts down the detoxification process, making the bad feelings go away. The worse the nutritional quality of your diet, the worse you will feel if you try to stop eating food for a few hours. You will only feel normal while your digestive tract is busy. You will feel better only if you over-consume calories, but of course, you won't be able to maintain a favorable weight. And when you are constantly eating and digesting food to avoid the discomfort of detoxification, weight gain is inevitable which itself leads to many other health problems such as heart disease and diabetes. We have become a nation of food addicts, driven to consume more calories than the body requires. I call this "toxic hunger".

Symptoms Of Toxic Hunger

- Headaches
- Weakness
- Stomach cramping
- Lightheadedness
- Esophageal spasms
- Growling stomach
- Irritability

Toxic hunger is a physical withdrawal from an unhealthy, low-micronutrient diet. Its symptoms are generally feelings that we have been taught to interpret as hunger. However, they are actually signs of your body's toxicity.

After years of eating a poor diet, detoxifying your body can be difficult. This is primarily because people often think that, since eating makes them feel better, the symptoms of detoxification they are feeling are actually hunger. This leads to one continuous eating binge all day. It is no wonder that 80 percent of Americans are overweight. Every few hours they are compelled to put something in their mouths. They may feel better temporarily from that chocolate-chip cookie or pretzel, but they never really get rid of the uncomfortable symptoms. This toxic hunger will recur whenever digestion ceases, not when an individual is truly hungry and has a biological need for calories. You become overweight because you feel the desire to eat so frequently. In the process, you lose your opportunity for a long life and a disease-free future.

When our diet contains too much salt, saturated fat, sweets, meat, and cheese, and not enough high-nutrient calories, we are even more likely to experience toxic withdrawal symptoms when digestion comes to an end. Your digestive tract is now actually being overworked almost all the time, you may not feel ill as frequently because these heavy foods take a long time to digest, but when digestion is done, the ill feelings can be quite powerful. Only a heavy meal or continuous eating keeps us comfortable.

Food addiction affects almost all of the American population. Once you address your addictions and use this knowledge to help yourself through the detoxification process, you will be able to more easily, efficiently, and pleasurably address your nutrient and caloric requirements. However, these sensations of toxic hunger make it almost impossible to stop a person from consuming too many calories by telling him to reduce portion sizes, cut back on calories, count points, or other typical dieting strategies. You can't easily stop overeating or expect a person to eat less food when they feel so bad when they do. Unless people are informed, they mistake the withdrawal symptoms they feel for hunger, or claim they have hypoglycemia and they simply can't help eating too frequently and too much.

Coping with the Toxic Change

It takes time to be comfortable with the changes in your life. It is not unusual to feel physically uncomfortable as you detoxify in the process of making over your body chemistry with a healthful diet. The more stimulating or harmful your prior habits, the worse you feel when you stop them. When breaking your addiction to salt, meat, dairy, saturated fat, processed foods and other substances you might feel headachy, fatigued, or even a little itchy or ill, but the good news is these symptoms rarely last longer than a week. However, if you are making the changes to nutritional excellence gradually, the uncomfortable symptoms should be minimized.

An important hurdle to achieving your ideal weight and excellent health is getting rid of your food addictions. After that occurs, you may feel like you have been freed from prison and will find it easier to move forward with the program and be one step closer to truly eating for health.

True Hunger Can Help You Be Healthy

Most Americans have never experienced *true hunger*. To learn to eat when you are truly hungry, you must know the difference between *toxic hunger* and *true hunger*. We think we are hungry when our stomach growls or we feel a little lightheaded. Think again: that is toxic hunger. It may take time but if you eat healthfully, your perception

54

of hunger will change and you simply will not be driven to overeat. When you eat right, you simply will not want so much food.

So the purpose of this prescription is to set you free from your food addictions and allow you to lose your toxic hunger. The food cravings will end and you will be able to stop overeating. Then, you will be back in contact with *true hunger*. When you achieve that, you will be able to accurately sense the calories you need to maintain your healthy and lean body.

I want to reiterate that as you adopt a high-nutrient eating-style by eating lots of healthy foods, it is common to go through an adjustment period in which you experience fatigue, weakness, lightheadedness, headaches, gas and other mild symptoms. This generally lasts less than a week. Don't panic or buy into the myth that to get relief you need more heavy or stimulating foods, such as high-protein foods, sweets or coffee.

True Hunger is Pleasurable

True hunger is not felt in the stomach or the head. When you eat healthfully and don't overeat, you eventually are able to sense true hunger and accurately assess your caloric needs. Once your body attains a certain level of better health, you will begin to feel the difference between true hunger and just eating due to desire, boredom, stress, or withdrawal symptoms. The best way to understand true hunger is to experience it for yourself. It has three primary characteristics:

1. **A sensation in your throat**
2. **Increased salivation**
3. **A dramatically-heightened taste sensation**

Being in touch with true hunger will help you reach your ideal weight. Plus, you will feel well all the time whether you eat, delay eating or skip a meal. Almost all of my patients who suffered with headaches and so-called "hypoglycemia" have gotten well permanently following my nutritional recommendations. The important point is they no longer are driven to overeat. Eating when you are truly hungry also makes eating food even more pleasurable because it enhances taste.

How True Hunger Works

This heightened taste sensation that accompanies true hunger gives us terrific feedback to inhibit overeating behavior so we can actually get more pleasure out of our diet. Delaying eating, to the point when true hunger is experienced, makes even ordinary foods taste great and extraordinary foods taste even better.

In our present toxic food environment, humans have lost the ability to connect with the body signals that tell them how much food they actually need. They have become slaves to withdrawal symptoms and eat all day long when there is no biological need for calories. Nature had a different plan. In an environment of healthy food choices, we would not feel any signals that it is time to eat after a meal until the hormonal and neurological messengers indicated the glycogen reserves in the liver were decreased and lean body mass would soon be used as an energy source. Your body has the beautifully orchestrated ability to give you the precise signals to tell you exactly how much to eat to maintain an ideal weight for your long-term health. These signals are what I call *true hunger*. This name also differentiates it from toxic hunger, which is what everyone else, including some medical textbooks, refers to simply as hunger. Most Americans have not felt true hunger since they were toddlers.

Feeding ourselves to satisfy true hunger cannot cause weight gain, and, if we only ate when truly hungry, it would be almost impossible for anyone to become overweight. True hunger is a signal for us to eat to maintain our muscle mass. Eating to satisfy true hunger does not put fat on our body. Excessive fat stores are developed only from eating outside of our body's true hunger demands.

When you get back in touch with true hunger, you will instinctually know how much to eat. When you exercise more, you will get more and more frequent hunger; when you exercise less, you will get much less hunger. Your body will become a precise calorie-measuring computer and steer you in the right direction just from eating the amount that feels right and makes food taste best. In order to achieve an ideal weight and consume the exact amount of calories to maintain a lean body mass that will prolong life, you must get rid of toxic hunger and get back in touch with true hunger. Eat when hungry, and don't eat when not hungry and you will never have to diet or be overweight again.

To lose more, eat more fiber and volume

When you are actively trying to lose weight, you should strive to satisfy your volume requirements. This may feel strange at first because you may not immediately feel satisfied by the higher volume of food. This is because you are accustomed to eating large quantities of high-calorie foods that cause a dopamine rush, a rush that low calorie foods don't deliver. However, your body will adjust, be less dependent on the dopamine surge in the brain, and will gradually become more and more satisfied with fewer calories. Give yourself time, and use the knowledge you have gained. Striving to fulfill your body's volume and nutrient requirements can help you resolve food cravings and your toxic hunger.

Just look at these three stomachs.

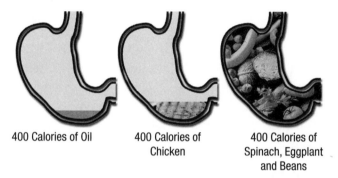

400 Calories of Oil   400 Calories of Chicken   400 Calories of Spinach, Eggplant and Beans

Each is filled with the same amount of calories, but one with oil, one with chicken and one with vegetables. The stomachs with the oil and chicken have a great deal of room in them, room that can enable you to easily overeat on calories. That's why filling your stomach with high-nutrient foods is so important to acquiring and maintaining a healthy weight. This leads us to a counterintuitive, but crucial rule: to lose more weight, and for better health, eat more high-volume, low calorie foods.

The trick to get you to desire fewer calories faster is to eat lots of these high-volume, high-nutrient foods. You are already familiar with these, but many of the foods that you have been incorporating into your diet because of their nutrient values are also great tools in meeting your volume requirements.

They include:

RAW VEGETABLES—lettuce, tomatoes, peppers, celery, anise, snow pea pods, carrots, beets, cucumbers, water chestnuts, green and red cabbage, onion, kale, collards, swiss chard, spinach, bok choy, parsley.

MOST FRESH FRUITS—melons, oranges, grapefruits, apples, kiwis, berries, papaya apples, apricots, blackberries, blueberries, raspberries, strawberries, grapes, mangoes, nectarines, peaches, pears, persimmons, pineapples, plums, tangerines.

COOKED GREEN VEGETABLES—Brussels sprouts, string beans, artichokes, asparagus, broccoli, Chinese cabbage, bok choy artichokes, asparagus, broccoli, Brussels sprouts, cabbage, celery, cucumber, kohlrabi, okra, peas, green peppers, snow peas, string beans, zucchini.

OTHER NON-GREEN VEGETABLES—mushrooms, eggplant, sun-dried tomatoes, onions, bean sprouts, cauliflower, spaghetti squash

BEANS AND LEGUMES—*(cooked, canned, or sprouted)* red kidney beans, adzuki beans, chickpeas, pinto beans, cowpeas, navy beans, cannelloni beans, soybeans, lentils, white beans, lima beans, pigeon peas, black-eyed peas, black beans, split peas.

Especially on holidays and days when you know that you will be around a lot of unhealthy foods, pre-fill with these high-nutrient, low-calorie foods. Never go to a party or event with an empty stomach. Eat a large salad with assorted raw vegetables and a bowl of vegetable soup before going to the places that may tempt your desire to eat unhealthily. Being healthy is about being in control. You must control your hunger, and the more low-calorie, high-volume foods you consume, the less high-calorie food you will be able to eat. When you increase these super-healthy foods in your diet, you will feel less temptation, and you will be in control of your food cravings and appetite. By eating mostly when you are truly hungry, food from nature will once again taste great. You will achieve great health and will always be at your ideal weight.

CHAPTER SEVEN

TOP NUTRITARIAN PRINCIPLES

Now that we have covered the most important aspects of the Eat Right America program, below is a top 10 list of most critical principles of becoming a Nutritarian.

1. **If it wasn't food 100 years ago, lay off it today!** 100 years ago, there were fewer heart attacks and strokes. There was less diabetes, obesity and cancer. Today these diseases eventually affect 90% of us. Today, over 60% of an average American's diet is processed foods— manufactured products void of nutrition and vitamins. Processed foods are also laden with salt and both saturated and trans fat which promote many diet-related chronic illnesses.

2. **H=N/C — Dr. Fuhrman's Health Equation**—Your long-term health is directly related to the amount of

Nutrients you get for each Calorie. The more "nutrient-dense" a food, the more powerful it is. The most nutrient-dense foods are fruits and vegetables, especially dark leafy greens which are the foods most missing in modern diets. Nutrient-dense foods contain vital nutrients, vitamin and minerals essential for preventing disease, boosting immunity, detoxifying the body and delivering permanent weight loss.

3. **Nutrition IS the Prescription!** Heart Disease, Type II Diabetes, Hypertension and many other conditions are directly related to poor dietary habits. The body has an incredible ability to heal itself when properly nourished and when we reduce the unhealthy foods we eat. For example, even patients on insulin for years can reduce and eventually eliminate medications as they lose weight and become healthy. Nutritional excellence is more effective than medications at resolving most medical problems while promoting a pleasurable, longer and more healthy life.

4. **If you want to lose weight — DON'T DIET!** 95% of all weight lost on most popular diets is regained. These diets are focused on counting and reducing carbohydrates, fats or protein as this is where calories come from. While many diets may produce short term weight loss, they cannot be maintained and therefore the weight returns. The only proven strategy for permanent

weight loss is to consume sufficient nutrients and fiber as a strategy for a lifetime of excellent health. This strategy will reduce your cravings for 'junk' food and curb the tendency to overeat. Then you will instinctually eat less calories, without struggle and without food addictions and cravings that have sabotaged your attempts in the past.

5. **Where's the Beef?** For years, the USDA Food Pyramid has suggested we consume beef and other animal products in order to get our protein. The USDA suggests approximately 600 calories of beef per day. Instead, remember that vegetables, beans and seeds are also high in protein, so there is no essential need to have animal products at every meal. In fact, broccoli has more protein per calorie than steak. Think about it… cows are vegan, as are gorillas and horses. Trying to lose weight or reduce your cholesterol? Think Greens for health and for building lean muscles. For great health we need to get more protein from nutrient-rich plant sources such as greens, beans, seeds and nuts and less from animal products.

6. **Milk?** An average cow produces 25 times more milk per year than just fifty years ago. Are cows getting bigger? Sure, we all need calcium for strong bones but calcium is just a small part of the story. Hundreds of other nutrients are also needed for healthy bones and intake of vegetables, not dairy is the best predictor of bone health.

Remember, green vegetables are not only higher in calcium than milk, but have the other accessory nutrients that build bones. For great health, we should get more calcium from nutrient rich plant sources such as greens, beans, seeds and nuts and less from dairy products. Our body needs thousands of discovered and undiscovered nutrients that work synergistically.

7. **Watch the Olive Oil!** One tablespoon of olive oil has 120 calories (all oils do). One-quarter cup has 500 calories. Healthy salads are definitely a way of life for people who want to lose weight or improve health. However, many of the benefits of a salad are lost when the calorie count is increased ten-fold with oil. Flavored vinegars, fruit and nut-based dressings are definitely the way to go. Nuts and seeds, not oil, have shown dramatic protection against heart disease. We need to get more of our fats from these wholesome foods and less from processed oils.

8. **If health came in a bottle — we'd all be healthy!** Natural, whole, plant-based foods are highly complex. It may never be possible to extract the precise symphony of nutrients found in fruits and vegetables and place it in a pill. So don't rely on pills and supplements to get your primary nutrition.

9. **Six-A-Day... Not The Way!** You have probably heard it's better to eat six small meals a day. That is not ideal.

You simply will not need to eat that frequently once your body is well nourished with micronutrients. The body can more effectively detoxify and enhance cell repair when not constantly eating and digesting. Eating right removes cravings and reduces the sensations driving us to eat too frequently and too much. For most people who follow a nutritarian diet-style, eating when truly hungry means eating three meals a day.

10. **Let Your Body Decide!** Nobody wants to hear that they have to give up all their favorite foods like pizza and ice cream. But wouldn't it be nice if over time your body actually preferred healthy foods over damaging ones? The body can change its taste and food preferences. As you consume larger and larger portions of health-promoting foods, your appetite for low-nutrient foods decreases and you gradually lose your addiction to sugar and fats. You learn to enjoy and prepare gourmet-tasting meals that are nutrient-rich. When this occurs, you have mastered becoming a Nutritarian!

We realize unhealthy foods can be very appealing and hard to resist. Please be patient with yourself as you start to eat right. As you switch your eating to healthy foods, you will lose your cravings for unhealthy foods and learn to eat when you are truly hungry. The best thing is your body will learn to love fresh fruits and vegetables because they taste so great and satisfying.

Becoming a Nutritarian is all about empowering you with the knowledge and support you need to once again get back in touch with the natural wisdom of your body.

Chapter Eight

NUTRIENT DENSITY SCORES

In this chapter, you will find extensive lists of nutrient/calorie-density scores grouped by category based on 'Aggregate Nutrient Density Index" (ANDI). Knowing which foods are high in nutrient density (and which are low) will make it easier to get the dramatic health benefits of eating more high-nutrient foods.

NOTE: *Calorie and Sodium data are provided for reference only. They are not related to ANDI scores. ANDI scores provide a relative ranking based on an equal amount of calories.*

	CALORIES	SODIUM	ANDI
VEGETABLES			
Kale, cooked (1.5 cups)	55	45	1000
Mustard Greens, cooked (1.5 cups)	32	34	1000
Turnip Greens, cooked (1.5 cups)	43	63	1000
Watercress, raw (3 cups)	11	42	1000
Collard Greens, cooked (1.5 cups)	74	46	1000

	CALORIES	SODIUM	ANDI
Kale, raw (1.5 cups)	50	43	896
Bok Choy, cooked (1.5 cups)	31	87	824
Spinach, raw (5 cups)	34	118	739
Broccoli Rabe, cooked (1.5 cups)	63	54	715
Chinese or Napa Cabbage, cooked (1.5 cups)	20	18	704
Spinach, cooked (1.5 cups)	62	189	697
Brussels Sprouts, cooked (1.5 cups)	84	49	672
Swiss Chard, cooked (1.5 cups)	52	470	670
Chinese or Napa Cabbage, raw (1.5 cups)	18	10	600
Chicory Greens, uncooked (1.5 cups)	62	122	591
Arugula, raw (5 cups)	25	27	559
Radish (6 items)	4	11	554
Cabbage, cooked (1.5 cups)	50	18	481
Bean Sprouts, uncooked (1 cup)	53	11	444
Cabbage, raw (1.5 cups)	32	24	420
Kohlrabi (1.5 cups)	54	40	393
Lettuce, Romaine (5 cups)	48	22	389
Broccoli, raw (1.5 cups)	45	44	376
Pepper, red, cooked (1.5 cups)	56	4	366
Radicchio (2 cups)	18	18	359
Broccoli, cooked (1.5 cups)	82	96	342
Turnips, cooked (1 item)	34	82	337
Carrots, cooked (1.5 cup)	81	136	336
Dandelion Greens, cooked (1.5 cups)	52	69	329

	CALORIES	SODIUM	ANDI
Pepper, red, raw (1.5 cups)	58	4	328
Chili Peppers, green, hot (1 item)	18	3	323
Escarole, raw (3 cups)	25	33	322
Mixed Baby Greens (5 cups)	37	35	300
Cauliflower, cooked (1.5 cups)	43	28	295
Cauliflower, raw (1.5 cups)	38	45	285
Pepper, green, raw (1.5 cups)	45	7	258
Artichoke, cooked (1 item)	60	114	244
Carrots, raw (1.5 cups)	75	126	240
Asparagus, cooked (1.5 cups)	59	38	234
Zucchini, raw (2.5 cups)	45	28	209
Tomato, cooked (1 cup)	43	26	190
Pepper, green cooked (1.5 cups)	57	4	181
Tomato, raw (1 item)	22	6	164
Jalapeno Peppers (0.13 cup)	7	0	164
Butternut Squash, cooked (1.5 cups)	122	12	156
Eggplant, cooked (1.5 cups)	50	1	149
Bamboo Shoots, canned (1 cup)	25	9	144
Okra, cooked (1.5 cups)	53	14	139
Mushrooms, raw (1.5 cups)	23	4	135
Celery (2 items)	11	64	135
Zucchini, cooked (1.5 cups)	43	8	132
Alfalfa Sprouts (1 cup)	10	2	130
Snow or sugar peas, raw (1.5 cups)	40	4	127

	CALORIES	SODIUM	ANDI
Mushrooms, cooked (1.5 cups)	66	5	119
Snow or sugar peas, cooked (1.5 cups)	101	10	113
Sun Dried Tomatoes (0.5 cup)	70	566	113
Lettuce, Iceberg (5 cups)	38	28	110
Rhubarb, cooked (1 cup)	25	5	106
Beets, cooked (1.5 cups)	112	196	97
Sweet Potato, cooked (1.5 cups)	378	134	83
Leeks, cooked (2 cups)	109	36	80
String Beans, cooked (1.5 cups)	65	6	75
Green Beans, cooked (2 cups)	87	2	74
Tomatillo (2 items)	22	1	72
Green Peas, cooked (1.5 cups)	202	7	70
Garlic Clove (1 item)	4	1	58
Cucumber (1 item)	45	6	50
Onions, cooked (0.33 cup)	31	2	50
Spaghetti Squash, cooked (1.5 cups)	63	42	49
Onions, raw (0.5 cup)	34	2	47
Acorn Squash, cooked (1.5 cups)	172	12	46
Corn, sweet, white, cooked (1.5 cups)	266	42	44
Potatoes, Flesh and skin, baked (1 item)	142	11	43
Parsnips (1.5 cups)	166	23	37
Potatoes, Flesh only, baked (1.5 cups)	170	9	31
Yams, cooked (1.5 cups)	266	20	23
Olives, (3 items)	36	408	24
Water chestnuts (1 cup)	70	11	19

	CALORIES	SODIUM	ANDI
FRUIT			
Strawberries (1.5 cups)	69	2	212
Blackberries (1.5 cups)	93	2	178
Plums (1.5 cups)	114	0	157
Raspberries (1.5 cups)	96	2	145
Lemon Juice (1teaspoon)	1	0	141
Blueberries (1.5 cups)	123	2	130
Papaya (1.5 cups)	82	6	118
Orange (1 item)	62	0	109
Grapefruit (1.5 cups)	144	0	102
Cantaloupe (1.5 cups)	82	38	100
Lime Juice (1 teaspoon)	1	0	99
Kiwi (2 items)	93	5	97
Watermelon (2.5 cups)	114	4	91
Peach (1 item)	38	0	73
Apple (1 item)	72	1	72
Tangerine, (2 items)	89	3	72
Cherries (1.5 cups)	137	0	68
Pineapple, (1.5 cups)	112	2	64
Figs, fresh (3 items)	111	2	62
Apricots fresh (4 items)	67	1	60
Mango, (1 item)	135	4	51
Prunes (0.25 cup)	102	1	47
Pears, (1 item)	96	2	46

	CALORIES	SODIUM	ANDI
Honeydew (1.5 cups)	96	48	45
Nectarine (1.5 cups)	91	0	41
Avocado, (half)	182	3	37
Cranberries, dried, sweetened (0.33 cup)	123	1	34
Grapes, (1.5 cups)	92	3	31
Banana, (1 item)	105	1	30
Apricots, dried, unsweetened (0.33 cup)	104	4	29
Figs, dried (0.25 cup)	124	5	25
Dates (0.25 cup)	125	1	19
Raisins (0.25 cup)	108	4	16

FRUIT/VEGETABLE JUICES

Vegetable Juice, low sodium (8 fluid ounces)	46	140	365
Vegetable Juice, regular (8 fluid ounces)	46	653	365
Carrot Juice (8 fluid ounces)	98	71	344
Tomato Juice, low sodium (8 fluid ounces)	41	24	342
Tomato Juice, regular (8 fluid ounces)	41	656	342
Pomegranate Juice, (8 fluid ounces)	150	10	193
Orange Juice (8 fluid ounces)	112	2	86
Cranberry Juice Cocktail (8 fluid ounces)	144	5	55
Apple Juice, unsweetened (8 fluid ounces)	117	7	16

	CALORIES	SODIUM	ANDI

BULK PRODUCTS

BEANS/LEGUMES

Lentils, boiled (1 cup)	230	4	104
Red Kidney Beans, boiled (1 cup)	225	2	100
Great Northern Beans, boiled (1 cup)	209	4	94
Adzuki Beans, boiled (1 cup)	294	18	84
Black beans, boiled (1 cup)	227	2	83
Black Eyed Peas, boiled (1 cup)	198	7	82
Hummus (0.5 cup)	218	298	70
Pinto Beans, boiled (1 cup)	245	2	61
Edamame (1 cup)	254	25	58
Split Peas, boiled (1 cup)	231	4	58
Chick Peas (Garbanzo), boiled (1 cup)	269	11	57
Lima Beans, boiled (1 cup)	216	4	46
Tofu (4 ounces)	69	9	37
Tempeh (4 ounces)	219	10	26

NUTS AND SEEDS

NUTS

Brazil (0.25 cup)	230	1	124
Pistachio Nuts, unsalted (0.25 cup)	183	3	48
Pecans (0.25 cup)	187	0	41
Almonds, unsalted (0.25 cup)	211	10	38

	CALORIES	SODIUM	ANDI
Peanuts, all types, unsalted (0.25 cup)	214	2	37
Walnuts (0.25 cup)	196	1	34
Hazelnuts or filberts (0.25 cup)	212	0	32
Cashew Nuts, unsalted (0.25 cup)	197	5	27
Pine Nuts or Pignolia (1 tablespoon)	58	0	26
Macadamia Nut, unsalted (0.25 cup)	241	1	17

Nut Butter

Tahini or Sesame Butter (2 tablespoons)	178	34	54
Almond (without salt) (2 tablespoons)	203	4	26
Cashew (without salt) (2 tablespoons)	188	5	26
Peanut (2 tablespoons)	188	147	26

Seeds

Sunflower (0.25 cup)	186	1	78
Sesame (0.25 cup)	206	4	65
Flax (2 tablespoons)	118	8	65
Pumpkin (0.25 cup)	187	6	52

GRAINS

Whole Grains

Oats, old fashioned, cooked (1 cup)	147	2	53
Barley, whole grain, cooked (1 cup)	193	5	43
Wild Brown Rice, cooked, (1 cup)	166	5	43

	CALORIES	SODIUM	ANDI
Brown Rice, cooked (1 cup)	216	10	41
Barley, pearled, cooked (1 cup)	193	5	32
Wheat Berries, cooked (1/2 cup)	150	0	25
Cornmeal, whole grain (0.25 cup)	110	11	22
Quinoa, cooked (1 cup)	222	13	21
Millet, cooked (1 cup)	250	3	19
Bulger, cooked (1 cup)	150	10	17

REFINED GRAIN PRODUCTS

	CALORIES	SODIUM	ANDI
Whole Wheat Flour (1/4 cup)	102	1.5	31
Whole Wheat Pasta, cooked (1 cup)	174	4	19
Oats, quick, cooked (1 cup)	147	2	19
White Pasta, cooked, (1 cup)	198	2	18
White Flour (1/4 cup)	114	1	18
Couscous, cooked (1 cup)	176	8	15
White Rice, long grain, cooked(1 cup)	216	10	12
Corn Pasta, cooked (1 cup)	176	0	10

BREADS/CRACKERS

	CALORIES	SODIUM	ANDI
Sprouted Grain Bread, (1 slice)	130	3	39
Whole Grain Bread (2 slices)	130	253	30
Whole Wheat Bread (2 slices)	130	265	25
Whole Wheat Bagel (1 item)	181	360	25
Tortilla, whole wheat (2 items, 67 grams)	180	500	21
Rye Bread (2 slices)	165	422	20
Plain Bagel (1 item)	195	379	18

	CALORIES	SODIUM	ANDI
White Bread (2 slices)	133	340	18
Tortilla, flour (2 items, 64 grams))	200	407	15
English Muffin, enriched (1 item)	134	264	13
Tortilla, corn, (2 items, 52 grams)	113	23	12
Rice Cake Cracker (7 pieces)	115	21	12
Saltines (5 items)	64	161	11
Graham crackers (2 1/2" sq.) (4 items)	118	169	8

CEREALS

Bran Flakes, (1 cup)	128	293	64
Granola (1 cup)	598	27	22

FISH

FRESH

Tuna, yellow fin*, cooked, dry heat (4 ounces)	158	53	46
Flounder, cooked, dry heat (4 ounces)	133	119	41
Sole, cooked, dry heat (4 ounces)	133	119	41
Salmon, pink, cooked, dry heat (4 ounces)	169	98	39
Mahi-Mahi*, cooked, dry heat (4 ounces)	124	128	39
Swordfish**, cooked, dry heat (4 ounces)	176	130	38
Trout, rainbow, wild, cooked, dry heat (4 ounces)	170	64	36
Snapper*, cooked, dry heat (4 ounces)	145	65	35

	CALORIES	SODIUM	ANDI
Haddock, cooked, dry heat (4 ounces)	127	99	35
Monkfish*, cooked, dry heat (4 ounces)	110	26	34
Cod, cooked, dry heat (4 ounces)	119	88	31
Grouper*, cooked, dry heat (4 ounces)	134	60	27
Tilapia, cooked, dry heat (4 ounces)	195	74	18

CANNED

Salmon (4 ounces)	158	628	42
Tuna*, in water (4 ounces)	145	428	36

SHELLFISH

Lobster*, cooked, (4 ounces)	111	431	43
Shrimp, cooked, (4 ounces)	112	254	38
Scallops, steamed (4 ounces)	120	478	24

Fish and shellfish may contain mercury and other pollutants[9]

** High level of mercury/pollutants

* Intermediate level of mercury/pollutants

MEAT

BEEF*

Ground Beef, 95% lean meat, (4 ounces)	194	73	29
Flank Steak, separable fat & lean, 0" fat (4 ounces)	213	63	27

	CALORIES	SODIUM	ANDI
Beef Top Round, separable fat & lean, 1/8" fat, (4 ounces)	231	46	22
Beef Skirt Steak, separable fat & lean, 0" fat (4 ounces)	289	104	21
Beef Top Sirloin, separable fat & lean, 1/8" fat, (4 ounces)	275	63	20
Ground Beef, 85% lean meat, (4 ounces)	284	82	20
Beef Tenderloin, separable fat & lean, 1/8" fat (4 ounces)	302	61	18
Beef Rib Eye Steak, separable fat & lean, 0" fat, (4 ounces)	300	60	18
Beef NY Strip Steak, separable fat & lean, 1/8" fat, (4 ounces)	317	76	16
Beef Prime Rib, separable fat & lean, 1/8" fat, (4 ounces)	437	70	12

cooking method-broiled

VEAL

	CALORIES	SODIUM	ANDI
Veal Loin, separable lean & fat, roasted (4 ounces)	246	105	17

BISON

	CALORIES	SODIUM	ANDI
Bison, Top Sirloin, separable lean only, broiled (4 ounces)	193	60	39
Bison, Chuck Roast, separable lean only, braised (4 ounces)	218	64	36

	CALORIES	SODIUM	ANDI

LAMB

	CALORIES	SODIUM	ANDI
Lamb, Leg, separable fat & lean, 1/8" fat, broiled (4 ounces)	274	76	20
Lamb, ground, broiled (4 ounces)	321	92	18
Lamb, Loin Chops, separable lean only, 1/8" fat, broiled (4 ounces)	337	88	16

PORK

	CALORIES	SODIUM	ANDI
Pork Tenderloin, separable lean & fat, roasted (4 ounces)	196	62	34
Pork Chops, center cut, separable lean, broiled (4 ounces)	272	65	24
Pork Loin, Whole, separable lean & fat, roasted (4 ounces)	281	67	23
Ham, Cured, Boneless, separable lean & fat, roasted (4 ounces)	276	1345	17
Pork Baby Back Ribs, separable lean & fat, roasted (4 ounces)	420	115	12
Bacon, cooked, (2 ounces)	302	1377	12

POULTRY

	CALORIES	SODIUM	ANDI
Chicken Breast, meat only, roasted (4 ounces)	187	84	27
Turkey, light meat only, roasted (4 ounces)	177	72	25
Turkey, dark meat only, roasted (4 ounces)	212	90	24
Chicken, dark meat only, roasted (4ounces)	232	105	17
Ground Turkey, broiled, (4 ounces)	266	121	16

	CALORIES	SODIUM	ANDI
Chicken Drumstick, meat & skin, roasted (4 ounces)	245	102	15
Chicken Wing, meat & skin, roasted (4 ounces)	329	93	11
Turkey Bacon, Cooked, (2 ounces)	217	1295	9

COLD CUTS

Turkey, white, rotisserie, deli cut (2 ounces)	64	680	33
Ham, 11% fat (2 ounces))	92	739	24
Roast Beef (2 ounces)	115	480	22
Bologna, beef and pork (2 ounces)	175	417	13

HOT DOGS AND SAUSAGE

Tofu Hot Dog (1 item)	163	330	23
Italian sausage, turkey (4 ounces)	179	1052	16
Hot Dog, turkey (1 item)	102	642	13
Italian sausage, pork (4 ounces)	390	1369	13
Bratwurst, (4 ounces)	337	962	13
Kielbasa, (4 ounces)	352	1220	11
Pepperoni (2 ounces)	264	1014	10
Hot Dog, beef (1 item)	148	513	8

	CALORIES	SODIUM	ANDI

DAIRY PRODUCTS & EGGS

BEVERAGES

Milk, Nonfat Skim (8 fluid ounces)	83	103	36
Milk, Low Fat 1% (8 fluid ounces)	105	127	28
Milk, Whole 3.3% (8 fluid ounces)	146	98	20
Chocolate Milk, low fat (8 fluid ounces)	158	152	19
Half & Half (2 tablespoons)	39	12	10
Heavy Whipping Cream (2 tablespoons)	104	11	2

CHEESE

Feta Cheese (2 ounces)	150	633	21
Cottage Cheese, low fat (1 cup)	163	918	18
Mozzarella Cheese, part skim (2 ounces)	144	351	16
Ricotta, part skim (1/2 cup)	170	154	16
Swiss cheese (2 ounces)	215	109	15
Parmesan (2 tablespoons)	43	153	15
Mozzarella Cheese, whole milk (2 ounces)	170	356	14
Gouda (2 ounces)	202	464	13
Provolone (2 ounces)	199	497	13
Cottage Cheese (1 cup)	216	850	13
Gruyere Cheese (2 ounces)	234	191	13
Muenster (2 ounces)	209	356	12
Blue Cheese (2 ounces)	200	791	12
Brie (2 ounces)	189	357	12
Monterey Jack (2 ounces)	211	304	12

	CALORIES	SODIUM	ANDI
Ricotta, whole milk (2 ounces)	214	103	11
Cheddar Cheese (2 ounces)	229	352	11
Cream Cheese, low fat (2 ounces)	139	178	8
Goat Cheese (2 ounces)	206	292	8
Cream Cheese (2 ounces)	193	182	4
Neufchatel, (2 ounces)	148	226	4

EGGS

Egg (1 item)	74	70	27

YOGURT

Plain Yogurt, non-fat, (1 cup)	80	115	30
Plain Yogurt, low-fat, (1 cup)	90	110	24
Tofu Yogurt (1 cup)	246	92	17
Plain Yogurt, whole milk (1 cup)	180	130	16
Fruit Yogurt, non fat, (1 cup)	130	100	16
Fruit Yogurt, low-fat, (1 cup)	130	95	15
Fruit Yogurt, whole milk (1 cup)	170	85	9

	CALORIES	SODIUM	ANDI
NON DAIRY MILK			
Soy Milk (8 fluid ounces)	125	132	33
Hemp Milk (8 fluid ounces)	100	5	27
Almond Milk (8 fluid ounces)	211	14	19
Rice Milk (8 fluid ounces)	120	86	10

PREPARED FOODS

CANNED FOODS			
Pumpkin, canned (0.5 cup)	42	6	372
Tomato Sauce, no salt added (1/4 cup)	20	20	248
Tomato Sauce, (1/4 cup)	20	321	248
Tomato Paste (2 tablespoons)	27	259	197
Tomato Paste, no salt added, (2 tablespoons)	27	32	197
Tomato, whole, diced, no salt added, (1 cup)	46	24	163
Tomato, whole, diced (1 cup)	41	307	163
Green Beans (3/4 cup)	18	236	76
Green Beans, no salt added, (3/4 cup)	18	2	76
Green Peas, (1/2 cup)	59	214	49
Green Peas, no salt added, (1/2 cup)	59	2	49
Yellow Corn, (1/2 cup)	66	175	28
Yellow Corn, no salt added (1/2 cup)	66	15	28
Peaches, halves, canned in own juice (1.5 cups)	164	15	29

	CALORIES	SODIUM	ANDI
Peaches halves, canned in light syrup (1.5 cups)	203	19	21
Peaches halves, canned in heavy syrup (1.5 cups)	291	24	16

FAST FOODS

Cheese Pizza (2 slices)	281	672	17
Biscuit w/ Egg & Bacon, fast food (1 item)	457	999	11
Fast Food Cheeseburger (1 item)	287	495	11
Fish Filet, Batter Coated, Fried (4 ounces)	263	603	10
French Fried Potatoes, fried in vegetable oil, fast food (2.5 ounces)	242	140	7

FROZEN DESSERTS

Vanilla Ice Cream (1 cup)	289	115	9
Sherbet, all flavors (1 cup)	213	68	9
Frozen Fruit & Juice Bar (1 item)	75	4	9
Vanilla Frozen Yogurt (1 cup)	221	125	8
Ice Pop or Popsicle (1 item)	42	7	0

	CALORIES	SODIUM	ANDI
SNACKS			
Dark Chocolate Candy Bar 45-59% cocoa (1.5 oz)	254	4	34
Milk Chocolate Candy Bar (1.5 oz)	235	35	21
Popcorn, air popped, no salt (4 cups)	122	1	16
Hard Pretzels, salted (60 grams) (10 items)	229	814	13
Fruit Roll Ups (1 item)	50	55	12
Chocolate Pudding (1 cup)	309	835	11
Potato Chips, salted (1 ounce)	152	168	11
Plain Granola Bar, (1 item)	115	72	11
Chocolate Sandwich Cookie with Creme Filling (3 items)	140	145	9
Toaster Pastry (1 item)	219	214	8
Fig Bar (2 items)	111	112	8
Popcorn, oil popped, no salt (4 cups) (44 grams)	229	1	8
Corn Puffs, cheese flavored (1 ounce)	157	298	8
Chocolate Chip Cookies, ready to eat (3 items)	147	89	7
Apple Pie, Prepared (1 slice)	411	327	6
Corn chips, plain (1 ounce)	153	179	6
Pound Cake (1 slice)	291	298	5
Chocolate Cake with Frosting (1 slice)	235	214	5

	CALORIES	SODIUM	ANDI

OTHER

BEVERAGES

Beer, 12 oz (12 fluid ounces)	139	14	7
Wine, (4 fluid ounces)	80	6	3
Cola (8 fluid ounces)	60	25	1

SPREADS/DIPS

Apple Butter (1 tablespoon)	93	8	3
All Fruit Preserves (1 tablespoon)	56	6	3
Margarine (1 tablespoon)	101	133	3
Jelly (1 tablespoon)	56	6	1
Butter (1 tablespoon)	102	82	1

SWEETENERS

Maple Syrup ((2 tablespoons)	104	4	4
Brown Sugar (1 tablespoon))	34	1	2
Corn Syrup (2 tablespoons)	128	28	1
Honey (1 tablespoon)	64	1	1
White Granulated Sugar (1 tablespoon)	49	0	0

OILS

Vegetable oil (1 tablespoon)	120	0	9
Olive Oil (1 tablespoon)	119	0	9

Appendix: How the ANDI was calculated

To determine the ANDI scores all known vitamins and minerals were added in. Nutrient data from Nutritionist Pro software for each food item was obtained for an equal calorie serving. Dr. Fuhrman included the following beneficial nutrients in the evaluation: calcium, carotenoids (beta carotene, alpha carotene, lutein, zeaxanthin lycopene) fiber, folate, glucosinolates ,iron, magnesium, niacin, resistant starch, selenium, sterols, vitamin B1 (thiamin) vitamin B2 (riboflavin), vitamin B6, vitamin B12, vitamin C, vitamin E, zinc, plus ORAC score (Oxygen Radical Absorbance Capacity). Nutrient quantities, which are normally in many different measurements (mg, mcg, IU) were converted to a percentage of their RDI so that a common value could be considered for each nutrient. Since there is currently no RDI for carotenoids, glucosinolates, or ORAC score, goals were established based on available research and current understanding of the benefits of these factors. The % RDI or Goal for each nutrient was added together to give a total. All nutrients were weighted equally with a factor of one except for the ORAC score, which was given a factor of 2 to partially account for undiscovered antioxidant nutrients. The sum of the food's total nutrient value was then multiplied by a fraction to make the highest number equal 1000 so that all foods could be considered on a numerical scale of 1 to 1000.

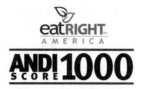

Please note: Eat Right America and Dr. Fuhrman are not claiming that ANDI* is the only factor to consider when devising the proper diet for you. However, it is likely the most important factor. There are some other scoring systems proposed and in use. The concern here is bias, results influenced by social, economic, or dietary agendas and preferences and not purely by science. In contrast, we made every effort to assure the ANDI was simply a mathematical formula that scores positive elements in food using dependable data, comprehensively, but without any preconceived or other promotional agenda. The results are mathematical and scientific, not opinion derived.

* *the ANDI food scoring system and its therapeutic application to medical conditions and health risk have a patent pending by Joel Fuhrman, MD and Kevin Leville of Eat Right America.*

CHAPTER NINE

HIGH NUTRIENT MENUS

Earlier, we mentioned that Eat Right America's Nutrition Prescription places people in one of three levels. In this chapter, we will do a comparison between a sample menu for each of the three levels against the Standard American Diet.

For your convenience, all items with an asterisk appear in Chapter 10, High Nutrient Recipes, beginning on page 99.

LEVEL ONE

Standard American Diet	Eat for Health Diet

BREAKFAST

Orange juice

Cheerios

Whole milk

LUNCH

Ham & cheese
sandwich on roll
w/ mayo

Potato chips

Coke

DINNER

Crackers w/
cheese spread

Spaghetti and
meatballs

Vanilla ice cream

*these items appear
in Chapter 10, High
Nutrient Recipes,
beginning on page 99.*

BREAKFAST

Fresh squeezed
orange juice

Oatmeal w/ blueber-
ries, apples & nuts

LUNCH

Turkey sandwich on
whole grain bread
w/ mixed greens
& tomato

Strawberries

Water

DINNER

Tasty Hummus w/
Baked Garlic Pita
Chips and raw
veggies*

Pasta w/ Roasted
Vegetables*

Creamy Banana
Walnut Ice Cream*

Nutritional Analysis	SAD	EFH
Calories	2011	1942
Protein	78	71
Carbohydrate	249	382
Fat	84	29
Cholesterol (mg)	337	20
Saturated fat	38	4
Fiber	15	54
Sodium (mg)	3660	1582
Vitamin C (mg)	183	603
B1, thiamine (mg)	2	3
B6, pyridoxine (mg)	1	3
Iron (mg)	23	23
Folate (mg)	409	802
Magnesium (mg)	148	491
Calcium	890	681
Zinc (mg)	9	9
Selenium (ug)	89	122
Alpha tocopherol (ug)	3	8
Beta carotene (ug)	120	10,339
Alpha Carotene (ug)	15	2,782
Lutein & Zeaxanthin (ug)	300	1,310
Lycopene (ug)	0	3,532
TOTAL NUTRIENT SCORE	**26**	**55**

LEVEL TWO

Standard American Diet	**Eat for Health Diet**

BREAKFAST

Blueberry muffin

Coffee/cream

LUNCH

Nachos w/ cheese

Cookies

DINNER

Iceberg lettuce salad
w/Italian dressing

Fried chicken

French fries

Corn

Cake

BREAKFAST

Blueberry Orange
Smoothie*

LUNCH

Bean Enchiladas*

Apple

DINNER

Mixed greens w/
Orange Cashew
Dressing*

Creole Chicken with
Broccoli and Spinach*

Brown Rice

Berry Cobbler*

*these items appear
in Chapter 10, High
Nutrient Recipes,
beginning on page 99.*

Nutritional Analysis	SAD	EFH
Calories	2030	1835
Protein	81	62
Carbohydrate	217	299
Fat	96	58
Cholesterol (mg)	277	36
Saturated fat	32	10
Fiber	15	55
Sodium (mg)	2889	440
Vitamin C (mg)	42	508
B1, thiamine (mg)	1	2
B6, pyridoxine (mg)	1	3
Iron (mg)	9	16
Folate (mg)	255	856
Magnesium (mg)	215	649
Calcium	746	617
Zinc (mg)	8	12
Selenium (ug)	59	74
Alpha tocopherol (ug)	5	17
Beta carotene(ug)	786	16,509
Alpha Carotene (ug)	5	4465
Lutein & Zeaxanthin (ug)	1257	11,978
Lycopene (ug)	795	10,471
TOTAL NUTRIENT SCORE	**19**	**71**

LEVEL THREE

Standard American Diet	Eat For Health Diet
BREAKFAST	**BREAKFAST**
Bagel w/ cream cheese	Lettuce, Banana & Cashew Wrap*
Orange juice	Pomegranate juice
LUNCH	**LUNCH**
Bacon ranch salad w/ crispy chicken	Romaine & spinach salad w/ Creamy Blueberry Dressing*
Ice tea	Fresh fruit & nut bowl
DINNER	**DINNER**
Chicken noodle soup	Raw veggies w/ Island Black Dip*
Grilled cheese sandwich	Dr. Fuhrman's Famous Anti-Cancer Soup*
Potato salad	Yummy, Quick & Easy Banana Oat Bars*
Brownie	

* these items appear
 in Chapter 10, High
 Nutrient Recipes,
 beginning on page 99.

Nutritional Analysis	SAD	EFH
Calories	2028	1985
Protein	67	70
Carbohydrate	212	335
Fat	105	58
Cholesterol (mg)	283	.2
Saturated fat	32	10
Fiber	11	62
Sodium (mg)	3832	1123
Vitamin C (mg)	167	495
B1, thiamine (mg)	1	2
B6, pyridoxine (mg)	.5	3
Iron (mg)	12	23
Folate (mg)	474	916
Magnesium (mg)	129	642
Zinc (mg)	5	10
Selenium (ug)	62	129
Alpha tocopherol (ug)	3	10
Beta carotene(ug)	1,557	36,165
Alpha Carotene (ug)	.02	6,089
Lutein & Zeaxanthin (ug)	.4	64,395
Lycopene (ug)	0	3,167
TOTAL NUTRIENT SCORE	**19**	**91**

CHAPTER TEN

HIGH NUTRIENT RECIPES

High-nutrient recipes taste great and are good for you! Those that follow are among the most healthful recipes in the world. Enjoy them, create variations, and start on the road to your optimal weight and health.

BREAKFASTS

BLUEBERRY ORANGE SMOOTHIE *Serves 2*

1 cup frozen blueberries

3 dates

2 oranges, peeled

1 banana

1 tablespoon ground flaxseeds

Blend in blender until smooth.

Per Serving:
Calories 207; Protein 2 g; Carbohydrate 49 g; Total Fat 2 g;
Saturated Fat 0.3 g; Cholesterol 0 mg; Sodium 3 mg

LETTUCE, BANANA, AND CASHEW WRAP *Serves 2*

2 teaspoons raw cashew butter, per leaf

12 romaine lettuce leaves

2 bananas , thinly sliced

Spread cashew butter on lettuce leaf, lay banana slices on
cashew butter and wrap lettuce around. A delicious and
healthy treat.

Per Serving:
Calories 312; Protein 8 g; Carbohydrate 39 g; Total Fat 17 g;
Saturated Fat 3 g; Cholesterol 0 mg; Sodium 15 g

CHOCOLATE CHERRY SMOOTHIE   *Serves 2*

4 ounces organic baby spinach

1/2 cup soy, hemp or almond milk

1/2 cup regular or cherry pomegranate juice

1 tablespoon natural cocoa powder

1 cup frozen cherries

1 banana

1 cup frozen blueberries

1/2 teaspoon vanilla extract

2 tablespoons ground flax seeds

In a high powered blender, liquefy the spinach with soy milk and juice. Add remaining ingredients and blend about 2 minutes until very smooth.

Per Serving:
Calories 259; Protein 6 g; Carbohydrate 52 g; Total Fat 5 g;
Saturated Fat 0.8 g; Cholesterol 0 mg; Sodium 75 mg

YUMMY, QUICK & EASY BANANA OAT BARS   *Serves 8*

2 cups quick oats (not instant)
1/4 cup chopped walnuts
1/2 cup shredded coconut
1/2 cup raisins or chopped dates
2 large ripe bananas, mashed
1/4 cup unsweetened applesauce, optional
1 tablespoon date sugar, optional

Preheat oven to 350 degrees. Mix ingredients together in a large bowl. Press dough in a 9"X 9" baking pan. Bake for 30 minutes. Cool on wire rack. When cool, slice into squares or bars and serve.

If you would like a sweeter, moister version of these bars, add the applesauce and date sugar.

Can be served for breakfast or as a healthy dessert.

Per Serving:
Calories 250; Protein 8 g; Carbohydrate 42 g; Total Fat 7 g;
Saturated Fat 2 g; Cholesterol 0 mg; Sodium 3 g

SOUPS

Fast Black Bean Soup   *Serves 5*

2 15-ounce cans black beans, no or low salt

2 cups frozen mixed vegetables

2 cups frozen corn

2 cups frozen chopped broccoli florets

2 cups carrot juice*

1 cup water

1 cup prepared black bean soup, no or low salt

1/4 cup chopped cilantro (optional)

1/8 teaspoon chili powder, or to taste

1 cup chopped fresh tomatoes

1 avocado, chopped or mashed (optional)

1/2 cup chopped green onions (optional)

1/4 cup raw pumpkin seeds (optional)

Combine black beans, mixed vegetables, corn, broccoli, carrot juice, water, soup, cilantro, and chili powder in a soup pot. Bring to a boil and simmer on low for 30 minutes. Stir in fresh tomatoes and heat through.

Serve topped with avocado, green onions, and pumpkin seeds if desired.

* Carrot juice may be made in a juice extractor. Fresh or bottled carrot juice is also sold in many health food stores.

Per Serving
Calories 403; Protein 25 g; Carbohydrate 80 g; Total Fat 2 g; Saturated Fat 0.4 g; Cholesterol 0 mg; Sodium 135 mg

DR. FUHRMAN'S FAMOUS ANTI-CANCER SOUP   *Serves 10*

1 cup dried split peas and/or beans

4 cups water

4 medium onions

6-10 medium zucchini

3 leek stalks

2 bunches kale, collards or other greens, chopped, tough stems and center ribs cut off and discarded

5 pounds carrots (4-5 cups juice)*

2 bunches organic celery (2 cups juice)*

2 tablespoons Dr. Fuhrman's VegiZest or Mrs. Dash

1 cup raw cashews

8 ounces mushrooms
(shiitake, cremini and/or oyster) chopped

Place the beans and water in a very large pot over low heat.

Add whole onions, whole zucchini and whole leeks to the pot along with chopped kale. Add carrot juice, celery juice and VegiZest (or Mrs. Dash).

Simmer mixture until onions, zucchini and leeks are soft, about 20 minutes. Remove the soft onions, zucchini, and leeks from the pot along with some of the soup liquid, being careful to leave the beans and some of the kale in the pot.

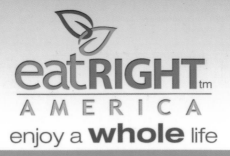

eatRIGHT™ AMERICA

enjoy a **whole** life

EAT ALL YOU WANT
- GREEN VEGETABLES
- COLORFUL VEGETABLES
- FRESH FRUIT
- BEANS / LEGUMES

EAT IN MODERATION
- WHOLE GRAINS / STARCHY VEGETABLES
- RAW NUTS AND SEEDS

EAT MORE ↑   EAT LESS ↓

- FISH
- NON-FAT DAIRY
- WILD MEAT AND FOWL

EAT RARELY
- RED MEAT
- REFINED GRAINS
- FULL-FAT DAIRY / CHEESE
- REFINED OIL / SWEETS

TOP 30 super foods

NUTRIENT SCORE

1.	Collard Greens, Mustard Greens, Turnip Greens	1000
2.	Kale	1000
3.	Watercress	1000
4.	Bok Choy	824
5.	Spinach	739
6.	Broccoli Rabe	715
7.	Chinese/Napa Cabbage	704
8.	Brussels Sprouts	672
9.	Swiss Chard	670
10.	Arugula	559
11.	Cabbage	481
12.	Romaine Lettuce	389
13.	Broccoli	376
14.	Red Pepper	366
15.	Carrot Juice	344
16.	Tomatoes and Tomato Products	164–300
17.	Cauliflower	295
18.	Strawberries	212
19.	Pomegranate Juice	193
20.	Blackberries	178
21.	Plums	157
22.	Raspberries	145
23.	Blueberries	130
24.	Oranges	109
25.	Cantaloupe	100
26.	Beans *(all varieties)*	57–104
27.	Seeds: Flaxseed, Sunflower, Sesame	52–78
28.	Pistachio Nuts	48
29.	Tofu	37
30.	Walnuts	34

**THE REVOLUTIONARY NUTRIENT SCORING SYSTEM
FOR MAXIMUM WEIGHT LOSS AND LIFELONG OPTIMAL HEALTH**

Using a blender or food processor, completely blend/puree the onions, zucchini, and leeks. Add more soup liquid and the cashews to the mixture, and blend in. Return the blended, creamy mixture back to the pot. Add the mushrooms and simmer another 30 minutes or until beans are soft.

* *Juice carrots and celery in a juice extractor. Fresh juiced organic carrots are necessary to maximize the flavor of this soup.*

Per Serving:
Calories 304; Protein 14 g; Carbohydrate 52 g; Total Fat 7 g; Saturated Fat 1 g; Cholesterol 0 mg; Sodium 135 mg

VEGETABLE AJIACO SOUP   *Serves 4*

2 cups fresh carrot juice

2 cups fresh celery juice

8 cups of water or low sodium vegetable broth

1 medium onion, diced

6 garlic cloves, chopped

1 malanga root

1 red pepper, cut into strips

4 cachucha peppers

4 ounces green beans

2 carrots, cut on the bias

2 medium potatoes, diced

2 kale leaves, chopped

this recipe developed by
ILLANSY RUIZ
from
Whole Foods Market

2 cups fresh corn kernels

1 cup tomato puree

2 tablespoons low sodium tamari

4 tablespoons nutritional yeast

2 cups fresh cooked beets, or canned if not available

3 cups baby spinach

2 ounces hemp seeds

black pepper

Mix the water or the broth with the carrot and the celery juice, then add remaining ingredients except baby spinach, beets, hemp seeds and black pepper. Simmer until vegetables are al dente. Add baby spinach and beets and heat until spinach is wilted. Stir in hemp seeds and season with black pepper to taste.

Per Serving
Calories 394; Protein 14 g; Carbohydrate 70 g; Total Fat 10 g;
Saturated Fat 1 g; Cholesterol 0 mg; Sodium 309 mg

GOLDEN AUSTRIAN CAULIFLOWER CREAM SOUP

Serves 4

1 head cauliflower, cut into florets

3 carrots, coarsely chopped

1 cup organic celery, coarsely chopped

2 leeks, coarsely chopped

2 tablespoons Dr. Fuhrman's VegiZest or other no salt seasoning

2 cups carrot juice

4 cups water

2 cloves garlic, minced

1/2 teaspoon nutmeg

1 cup raw cashews

5 cups kale leaves, chopped (organic baby spinach may also be used)

Cover and simmer all ingredients, except cashews and kale or spinach, for 15 minutes or until just tender.

If kale is being used steam until tender.

Blend 2/3 of soup vegetables and liquid with cashews until smooth and creamy. Add back to the remaining chunky vegetables and stir in steamed kale or spinach. Spinach will wilt in hot soup.

Per Serving
Calories 351; Protein 12 g; Carbohydrate 45 g; Total Fat 17 g;
Saturated Fat 3 g; Cholesterol 0 mg; Sodium 164 mg

SALAD DRESSINGS

RUSSIAN FIG DRESSING   *Serves 2*

2 tablespoons black fig or balsamic vinegar

1/4 cup pasta sauce, no or low salt

3 tablespoons raw almond butter or 1/3 cup raw almonds

Mash all ingredients together with a fork to blend.

Per Serving:
Calories 118; Protein 3 g; Carbohydrate 13 g; Total Fat 7 g;
Saturated Fat 0.8 g; Cholesterol 0 mg; Sodium 4 mg

CAESAR SALAD DRESSING/DIP   *Serves 3*

3 cloves garlic, roasted*

1/2 cup soy, hemp or almond milk

1/4 cup raw cashew butter or 1/2 cup raw cashews

1 tablespoon fresh lemon juice

1 tablespoon nutritional yeast (optional)

1 1/2 teaspoons Dijon mustard

dash black pepper

Roast garlic. Remove skins and blend with the rest of the ingredients in a high powered blender until creamy and smooth.

To roast garlic; break the cloves apart. Leave the papery skins on. Roast at 350 degrees for about 25 minutes until mushy.

Per Serving:
Calories 154; Protein 6 g; Carbohydrate 9 g; Total Fat 11 g;
Saturated Fat 2 g; Cholesterol 0 mg; Sodium 86 mg

SUN DRIED TOMATO VINAIGRETTE OR MANGO VINAIGRETTE

1/4 cup sun dried tomatoes, drained

1 1/2 tablespoons white wine vinegar

1/2 clove of fresh minced garlic

1 1/2 tablespoons fresh minced shallots

1 teaspoon ground cumin

1/2 teaspoon dried basil

1/2 cup spinach juice

1 1/2 teaspoons date sugar

1/3 cup tomato puree

1/4 cup chopped parsley

1/2 cup raw cashews

this recipe developed by
ILLANSY RUIZ
from
Whole Foods Market

Place all the ingredients into the food processor except the cashews. Blend until smooth and then add the cashews. Continue to blend until creamy.

Note: To make mango vinaigrette add 3/4 cup of mango puree to the Sun Dried Tomato Vinaigrette.

Per Serving:
Calories 135; Protein 4 g; Carbohydrate 11 g; Total Fat 9 g;
Saturated Fat 2 g; Cholesterol 0 mg;

CASHEW ORANGE DRESSING/DIP   *Serves 2*

2 oranges peeled and quartered

3 tablespoons raw cashew butter or

1/3 cup raw cashews

2 tablespoons blood orange or other fruity vinegar

1/2 teaspoon lemon juice (optional)

orange juice (optional)

Blend until smooth, adding orange juice if too thick.

Per Serving:
Calories 127; Protein 3 g; Carbohydrate 15 g; Total Fat 7 g;
Saturated Fat 1 g; Cholesterol 0 mg; Sodium 3 g

MAIN DISHES

CREOLE CHICKEN
WITH BROCCOLI AND SPINACH   *Serves 4*

nonstick cooking spray

1-2 skinless, boneless chicken breast halves,
thin sliced crosswise

1 1/2 cups chopped organic celery

1 cup chopped canned tomatoes, (no salt)

10 ounces frozen broccoli, thawed

1 cup chili sauce (low salt)

1/4 cup chopped onion

1 large green pepper, chopped

2 cloves garlic, minced

1 tablespoon chopped fresh basil or 1 teaspoon dried

1 tablespoon chopped fresh parsley or
1 teaspoon dried

1/8 - 1/4 teaspoon dried crushed red pepper

4-5 cups fresh baby spinach

Spray deep nonstick skillet with cooking spray and heat.
Cook thin strips of chicken on medium high, turning
occasionally, for 3-5 minutes until no longer pink.

Add remaining ingredients except spinach, bring to a

boil and reduce heat to medium. Simmer covered for 15 minutes or until vegetables are tender. Add spinach and continue cooking until wilted.

Serve over brown rice.

Per Serving:
Calories 359; Protein 23 g; Carbohydrate 65 g; Total Fat 3 g; Saturated Fat 0.6 g;
Cholesterol 34 mg; Sodium 148 mg

EGGPLANT ROLANTINI   *Serves 4*

1 large eggplant

1 cup coconut milk

1 collard green leaf, diced

1 medium zucchini, diced

1 carrot, diced

1/2 onion, diced

2 sushi nori sheets, diced

dash of saffron

16 ounces organic firm tofu (*Whole Foods Market 365 Brand* works great)

1 tablespoon nutritional yeast

dash cayenne pepper

1 tablespoon dry oregano

1 1/2 cups organic tomato sauce, low sodium

4 slices vegan low fat cheese (optional)

this recipe developed by
ILLANSY RU
from
Whole Foods Market

Preheat the oven to 325° F.

Slice the eggplant length wise about 1/4 inch thick. Marinate in 1/2 cup of the coconut milk with some fresh ground black pepper. Let set for 10 minutes.

Place the eggplant on an ungreased baking sheet and bake for 10 minutes until lightly browned. Saute the vegetables with the remaining coconut milk. Add the saffron and let cook for 10 minutes until vegetables are translucent.

Crumble the tofu until it looks like scrambled eggs and add to the vegetables. Add the pepper, oregano and nutritional yeast and cook for another 5 minutes over low heat.

Once the eggplant has cooled, put several spoonfuls of the cooked vegetable mixture on one end and roll, keeping the filling inside. Repeat this with all eggplant slices.

Place the eggplant rolls into a ceramic baking dish and cover with tomato sauce and shredded cheese. Bake at 325° F for about 10 minutes or until heated through.

Per Serving:
Calories 384; Protein 9 g; Carbohydrate 45 g; Total Fat 21 g;
Saturated Fat 13 g; Cholesterol 0 g; Sodium 68 g

PASTA WITH ROASTED VEGETABLES, TOMATOES AND BASIL

Serves 6

non-stick cooking spray

2 red bell peppers, cut into 1/2 inch pieces

1 medium eggplant, unpeeled,
cut into 1/2 inch pieces

1 large yellow crookneck squash,
cut into 1/2 inch pieces

1 1/2 cups 1/2 inch pieces peeled butternut squash

2 tablespoons olive oil, divided

1 pound penne pasta, preferably whole wheat

2 medium tomatoes, cored, seeded, diced

1/2 cup chopped fresh basil or 1 1/2 tablespoons dried

2 tablespoons balsamic vinegar or 1 tablespoon fresh
lemon juice

2 cloves garlic, minced

Preheat oven to 450 degrees. Spray large roasting pan
with nonstick spray. Combine red bell peppers, eggplant,
yellow squash, and butternut squash in prepared pan.
Drizzle with 1 tablespoon olive oil and toss to coat. Roast
until vegetables are tender and beginning to brown,
stirring occasionally, about 25 minutes.

Meanwhile, cook pasta and drain, reserving 1/2 cup
cooking liquid.

Combine pasta, roasted vegetables, tomatoes, basil in large bowl. Add remaining tablespoon of oil, vinegar and garlic. Toss to combine. Add cooking liquid by tablespoons to moisten, if desired.

Per Serving:
Calories 365; Protein 14 g; Carbohydrate 71 g; Total Fat 6 g; Saturated Fat 1 g; Cholesterol 0 mg; Sodium 14 mg

BEAN ENCHILADAS   *Serves 6*

1 green pepper, chopped

1/2 cup sliced onion

8 ounce can tomato sauce, no salt added

2 cups canned or cooked pinto or black beans

1 cup corn, frozen, thawed

1 tablespoon chili powder

1 teaspoon cumin

1 teaspoon onion powder

1 tablespoon chopped cilantro

1/8 teaspoon cayenne pepper (optional)

6-8 corn tortillas

Saute green pepper and onion in 2 tablespoons of the tomato sauce, until tender. Stir in the remaining tomato sauce, beans, corn, seasonings and cilantro and simmer for 5 minutes. Spoon about 1/4 cup of the bean mixture on each tortilla and roll up. They can be eaten as is or baked at 375 degrees for 15 minutes.

Per Serving:
Calories 185; Protein 9 g; Carbohydrate 37 g; Total Fat 2 g;
Saturated Fat 0.3 g; Cholesterol 0; Sodium 32 mg

SIDE DISHES

CALIFORNIA CREAMED KALE   *Serves 4*

2 bunches kale, leaves removed from tough stems and chopped

1 cup raw cashews

1 cup soy milk

4 tablespoons onion flakes

1 tablespoon Dr. Fuhrman's VegiZest (optional)

Place kale in a large steamer pot. Steam 10-20 minutes until soft.

Meanwhile, place remaining ingredients in a high-powered blender and blend until smooth.

Place kale in colander and press with to remove some of the excess water. In a bowl, coarsely chop and mix kale with the cream sauce.

Note: Sauce may be used with broccoli, spinach, or other steamed vegetables.

Per Serving:
Calories 269; Protein 12 g; Carbohydrate 25 g; Total Fat 16 g; Saturated Fat 3 g; Cholesterol 0 mg; Sodium 78 mg

Asparagus Vinaigrette   *Serves 4*

1/3 cup black fig or balsamic vinegar

1 tablespoon Dr. Fuhrman's VegiZest
or other no salt seasoning

3 tablespoons water

1 tablespoon Dijon mustard

1 tablespoon chopped fresh marjoram
or 1 teaspoon dried

1 teaspoon minced garlic

1 tablespoon almond butter

1 tablespoon ketchup, low sodium

2 pounds asparagus, tough ends trimmed,
then cut on diagonal into 2-inch pieces

1 small red bell pepper, very thinly sliced

1/2 cup pecans, toasted * and chopped (optional)

Boil vinegar in heavy small saucepan over medium heat until reduced by half, about 3 minutes. Pour vinegar into large bowl.

Combine water with no salt seasoning. Whisk into vinegar along with mustard, marjoram, garlic, almond butter and ketchup. Set dressing aside.

Sauté asparagus in small amount of water, stirring over high heat for 3 minutes, then cover and steam for 1 minute. Remove to a bowl.

In same pan, sauté bell peppers in a small amount of water for 1 minute.

Add asparagus and bell peppers to dressing; toss to blend well. Sprinkle with pecans if desired.

Note: Lightly toast pecans in a 200 degree oven for 3 minutes.

Per Serving:
Calories 104; Protein 7 g; Carbohydrate 14 g; Total Fat 3 g;
Saturated Fat 0.3 g; Cholesterol 0 mg; Sodium 108 mg

LEMON ZEST SPINACH   *Serves 4*

1 1/4 pounds fresh organic spinach or 4 bags organic baby spinach

6 cloves garlic, minced

5 tablespoons pine nuts

3 teaspoons lemon juice

1 teaspoon olive oil

1/2 teaspoon lemon zest

Steam spinach and garlic until spinach is just wilted.

Place in bowl and toss in remaining ingredients.

Per Serving:
Calories 123; Protein 6 g; Carbohydrate 8 g; Total Fat 9 g;
Saturated Fat 1 g; Cholesterol 0 mg; Sodium 113 mg

Tasty Hummus   *Serves 4*

>   1 cup cooked or canned garbanzo beans
>   (low or no salt), reserving liquid
>
>   1/4 cup bean liquid or water
>
>   1/4 cup raw unhulled sesame seeds
>
>   1 tablespoon lemon juice
>
>   1 tablespoon Dr. Fuhrman's VegiZest
>   or other no salt seasoning
>
>   1 teaspoon Bragg Liquid Aminos
>   or low sodium soy sauce
>
>   1 teaspoon horseradish (optional)
>   1 small clove garlic, chopped

Blend all ingredients in a high powered blender until creamy smooth.

This is a great spread or dip for raw and lightly steamed vegetables.

Per Serving:
Calories 127; Protein 6 g; Carbohydrate 15 g; Total Fat 6 g;
Saturated Fat 0.7 g; Cholesterol 0 mg; Sodium 79 mg

GARLIC PITA CHIPS   *Serves 2*

    2 whole grain pita bread
    olive oil spray
    1/8 teaspoon garlic powder

Preheat oven to 375 degrees. Cut each pita bread in half
horizontally. Spray pita halves lightly with olive oil and
sprinkle with garlic powder. Cut each half into four sec-
tions to form triangles. Place on baking sheet and bake
for 6 – 8 minutes or until lightly browned. Serve with
salsa or hummus.

Per Serving:
Calories 85; Protein 3 g; Carbohydrate 18 g; Total Fat 0.8 g;
Saturated Fat 0 g; Cholesterol 0 mg; Sodium 170 mg

GUACAMOLE   *Serves 4*

    2 medium size avocados, mashed
    1/4 cup yellow onions, diced
    2/3 cup roma tomatoes, diced
    1 clove fresh minced garlic
    1 minced jalapeno, without seeds
    1 tablespoon lemon juice
    1/2 teaspoon ground cumin
    1 tablespoon spinach juice
    1/4 cup chopped cilantro
    1 dash of black pepper

*this recipe
developed by*
ILLANSY RUIZ
from
Whole Foods
Market

Place all ingredients into a large bowl, and mix well.

Per Serving:
Calories 199; Protein 5 g; Carbohydrate 15 g; Total Fat 15 g;
Saturated Fat 3 g; Cholesterol 0 mg; Sodium 14 mg

BROCCOLI, KALE AND ROASTED GARLIC SALAD   *Serves 4*

6 cups broccoli, chopped

6 kale leaves

1 head garlic, roasted*

1/2 teaspoon of chili flakes

1 tablespoon flax seed oil

1/2 teaspoon lemon juice

1 tablespoon of nutritional yeast

this recipe developed by
ILLANSY RUIZ
from
Whole Foods Market

Steam broccoli for three minutes. Steam kale for 1 minute and chop. Roast garlic and remove skins. In a large bowl, combine broccoli, kale and roasted garlic. Mix together remaining ingredients and add to broccoli mixture.

* *To roast garlic: Break cloves apart, leaving papery skins on. Roast at 350 degrees for about 25 minutes or until mushy.*

Per Serving:
Calories 75; Protein 5 g; Carbohydrate 15 g; Total Fat 1 g;
Saturated Fat 0 g; Sodium 61 g

Island Black Bean Dip   *Serves 4*

1 15-ounce can no salt added black beans, drained

2 teaspoons no-salt salsa

1/4 cup scallions, minced

1 1/2 tablespoons blood orange or
other fruity vinegar

2 tablespoons Dr. Fuhrman's MatoZest or other
no salt seasoning

2 tablespoons minced red onion

1/2 cup finely diced mango

1/4 cup diced red pepper

1 tablespoon fresh, minced cilantro,
for garnish (optional)

Remove 1/4 cup of the black beans and set aside. Place remaining beans in a blender or food processor. And salsa, scallions, vinegar and Dr. Fuhrman's MatoZest. Puree until relatively smooth. Adjust seasonings to taste. Transfer to a bowl and add the red onion, mango and red bell pepper. Mix well and chill for 1 hour. Serve garnished with optional cilantro and raw veggies, unsalted, oil-free baked pita.

Per Serving:
Calories 106; Protein 6 g; Carbohydrate 21 g; Total Fat 0 g;
Saturated Fat 0 g; Cholesterol 0 mg; Sodium 39 mg

DESSERTS

CREAMY BANANA WALNUT ICE CREAM   *Serves 2*

    2 ripe bananas, frozen*
    1/3 cup vanilla soy, hemp or almond milk
    1/2 ounce walnuts

Blend all ingredients together in high powered blender
until smooth and creamy.

** Note: Freeze ripe bananas at least 24 hours in advance. To freeze
bananas, peel, cut in thirds and wrap tightly in plastic wrap.*

Per Serving:
Calories 172; Protein 4 g; Carbohydrate 30 g; Total Fat 6 g;
Saturated Fat 1 g; Cholesterol 0 mg; Sodium 23 mg

BERRY COBBLER   *Serves 2*

    1 banana, sliced
    1 cup frozen mixed berries
    dash cinnamon
    few drops vanilla extract

Put banana into a small microwave safe bowl. Add frozen
berries on top. Sprinkle with cinnamon and add vanilla.
Microwave for about 2 minutes. Serve warm.

Per Serving:
Calories 79; Protein 1 g; Carbohydrate 20 g; Total Fat 0 g;
Saturated Fat 0 g; Cholesterol 0 mg; Sodium 2 mg

WILD APPLE CRUNCH   *Serves 8*

    6 apples, peeled and sliced
    3/4 cup chopped walnuts
    8 dates, chopped
    1 cup currants or raisins
    3/4 cup water
    1/2 teaspoon cinnamon
    1/4 teaspoon nutmeg
    juice of 1 orange

Preheat oven to 375 degrees.

Combine all ingredients except the orange juice. Place in a baking pan and drizzle the orange juice on top.

Cover and bake at 375 degrees for about one hour until all ingredients are soft, stirring occasionally.

Note: You can also simmer this in a covered pot for 30 minutes on top of the stove, stirring occasionally.

Per Serving:
Calories 207; Protein 5 g; Carbohydrate 37 g; Total Fat 7 g;
Saturated Fat 0.7 g; Cholesterol 0 mg; Sodium 4 mg

QUINOA PUDDING: *Serves 4*

1 cinnamon stick

1/2 cup quinoa

2 1/2 cup water

2 cloves

1 1/4 cup vanilla soy milk

zest of 1 orange

1 1/4 cups coconut milk

1 tablespoon ground flax seeds mixed with
3 tablespoons water

1 tablespoon Port

1 tablespoon date sugar

ground cinnamon

*this recipe
developed by*
ILLANSY RUIZ
from
Whole Foods
Market

Combine cinnamon, quinoa, water and cloves and cook over medium heat until thickened. Add soy milk and orange zest and simmer until liquid is evaporated.

Add coconut milk, stirring constantly until mixture thickens. Combine flax seeds and water mixture with Port and date sugar. Add to quinoa.

Garnish with cinnamon.

Per Serving:
Calories 283; Protein 8 g; Carbohydrate 24 g; Total Fat 18 g;
Saturated Fat 14 g; Cholesterol 0 mg; Sodium 59 mg

REFERENCES

1. Keehan, S. et al. "Health Spending Projections Through 2017, Health Affairs Web Exclusive W146: 21 February 2008.

2. Gardner CD, Coulston A, Chatterjee L, et al. The effect of a plant-based diet on plasma lipids in hypercholesterolemic adults: a randomized trial. Ann Intern Med. 2005;142(9):725-733. Tucker KL, Hallfrisch J, Qiao N, et al. The combination of high fruit and vegetable and low saturated fat intakes is more protective against mortality in aging men than is either alone: the Baltimore Longitudinal Study of Aging. J Nutr. 2005;135(3):556-561.

3. Fuhrman J, Sarter B, Campbell TC. Effect of a high-nutrient diet on long-term weight loss: a retrospective chart review. Altern Ther Health Med 2008;14(3):48-53.

4. Svendsen M, Blomhoff R, Holme I, Tonstad S. The effect of an increased intake of vegetables and fruit on weight loss, blood pressure and antioxidant defense in subjects with sleep related breathing disorders. Euro J Cl in Nutr.2007;61:1301–1311. Ello-Martin JA, Roe LS, Ledikwe JH, et al. Dietary energy density in the treatment of obesity: a year-long trial comparing 2 weight-loss diets. Am J Clin Nutr. 2007; 85(6):1465-1477. Howard BV,Manson JE, Stefanick ML, et al. Low-fat dietary pattern and weight change over 7 years: the Women's Health Initiative Dietary Modification Trial.JAMA. 2006; 295(1):39-49.

5. Liu RH. Potential synergy of phytochemicals in cancer prevention: mechanism of action. J Nutr. 2004;134(12 Suppl):3479S-3485S. Weiss JF,Landauer MR. Protection against ionizing radiation by antioxidant nutrients and phytochemicals. Toxicology 2003;189(1-2):1-20. Carratù B, Sanzini E. Biologically-active phytochemicals in vegetable food. Ann Ist Super Sanita.2005; 41(1):7-16.

6. Hu FB. Plant-based foods and prevention of cardio-vascular disease: an overview. Am J Clin Nutr. 2003 Sep;78(3 Suppl):544S-551S. Campbell TC, Parpia B, Chen J. Diet, lifestyle, and the etiology of coronary artery disease:the Cornell China study. Am J Cardiol 1998 Nov 26;82(10B):18T-21T. Fujimoto N, Matsubayashi K, Miyahara T, et al. The risk factors for ischemic heart disease in Tibetan highlanders. Jpn Heart J. 1989 Jan;30(1):27-34. Tatsukawa M, Sawayama Y, Maeda N, et al. Carotid atherosclerosis and cardiovascular risk factors: a comparison of residents of a rural area of Okinawa with residents of a typical suburban area of Fukuoka, Japan.Atherosclerosis 2004;172(2):337-343.

7. Hu FB, Willett WC. Optimal diets for prevention of coronary heart disease. JAMA 2002 Nov 27;288(20):2569-2578. Esselstyn CB. Resolving the Coronary Artery Disease Epidemic Through Plant-Based Nutrition. 2001 Autumn;4(4):171-177.

8. Lawton CL, Burley VJ, Wales JK, Blundell JE. Dietary fat and appetite control in obese subjects: weak effects on satiation and satiety. Int J Obes Metab Disord 1993;17(7):409-416. Blundell JE, Halford JC. Regulation of nutrient supply: the brain and appetite control Proc Nutr Soc 1994;53(2):407-418. Stamler J, Dolecek TA. Relation of food and nutrient intakes to body mass in the special intervention and usual care groups on the Multiple Risk factor Intervention Trial. Am J Clin Nutr 1997;65(1 Suppl):366S-373S.

9. US Department of Health & Human Services, US Food & Drug Administration, Mercury Levels in Commercial Fish and Shellfish, http://www.fda.gov/ Food/FoodSafety/Product-SpecificInformation/Seafood/ FoodbornePathogensContaminants/Methylmercury/ ucm115644.htm date accessed August 18. 2009. Hightower JM, Moore D. Mercury Levels in high-end consumers of fish. Environmental Health Perspectives 2003; 111(4):604-908. Mahaffey KR, Clickner RP, Bodurow CC. Blood organic mercury and dietary mercury intake: National Health and Nutrition Examination Survey, 1999 and 2000. Env. Health Persp 2004; 112(5):562-570.

You Can *Personalize* Your Nutritarian Plan with…

EAT RIGHT AMERICA'S
NUTRITION PRESCRIPTION™

ERA's Nutrition Prescription is the nation's ONLY on-line, personalized, eating plan designed specifically to ensure *you* get the nutritional guidance *you* need to **enjoy a whole life.**

Every year, thousands of patients travel from all over the world to Dr. Fuhrman for a costly, medical consultation that can dramatically extend their life and forever change their health destiny. They include famous actors and actresses, singers, sport stars, corporate executives and people just like you. Their health concerns range from overweight to diabetes, heart disease, hypertension, asthma, allergies, autoimmune diseases and a host of other conditions. In every case, **Nutrition Is The Prescription**. Eat Right America's Nutrition Prescription has computerized this extensive evaluation and Dr. Fuhrman's insightful recommendations and made it affordable for all.

A TWO-YEAR STUDY OF THE HIGH NUTRIENT DIET PRODUCED AN AVERAGE WEIGHT LOSS OF 53 POUNDS.

Nutrition Prescription is now available from the privacy of your home for a remarkable price of
only $14.95.

After a ten minute on-line survey the Nutrition Prescription will produce:

- A Personal Eating Assessment.
- A Personal Disease Risk Evaluation
- A Personal Eating Plan
- A Personal Fitness Plan
- Customized nutritional recommendations that meet your unique needs
- 28 Days of Personal Emails to Support Your Plan
- 30 Days Free Access to the Eat Right America Community Website

For information on how to get started, visit:

www.EatRightAmerica.com/handbook
or call
1-877-525-8384